# SANE ASYLUMS

"*Sane Asylums* is a brilliant stroll through medi~~ ~~ 'g that homeopathic physicians were more than a h~~ ~~ time. The homeopathic mental health inst~~ ~~ hat is, they integrated homeopathic ~~ ~~ al exercise, play therapy, and respect ~~ ~~. In terms of mental health care, we can ~~ ~~ the 'good old days' in this medical specialty."

DA~~ ~~., MPH, CCH, AUTHOR OF
*THE HOMEOPATHIC REVOLUTION*

"Mental health professionals and patients alike can take heart from this thoroughly documented description of natural cures for mental illness at the turn of the last century. The actual cures came from the timeless science of homeopathy, whose safe and effective medicines remain in use today. In fact, we can still implement the same protocols that Jerry Kantor describes in *Sane Asylums,* complete with specific medicines for common diagnoses. Both scholarly and entertaining, *Sane Asylums* provides solid support for a more sane approach to mental illness today."

BURKE LENNIHAN, RN, CCH, CLASSICAL HOMEOPATH AND
AUTHOR OF *YOUR NATURAL MEDICINE CABINET*

"In *Sane Asylums,* Jerry Kantor digs into the past to reveal a surprising history, one that challenges current societal beliefs. The most joyful chapter in this book tells of 'baseball therapy' practiced at Middletown State Homeopathic Hospital for the Insane, with the Asylums, as the hospital's team was known, posting a surprisingly good record in competition with other local New York baseball teams. You read this and can't help but ask yourself, what does this reveal about our mental health care today?"

ROBERT WHITAKER, AUTHOR OF *MAD IN AMERICA*

"Jerry Kantor's book is an amazing historical document that also provides insight into what can be done to improve the lives of those struggling with mental illness today. Homeopathy *can* work miracles. It is imperative that more people realize this at a time when modern medicine is increasingly harming rather than helping us."

AMY L. LANSKY, PH.D., AUTHOR OF
*IMPOSSIBLE CURE: THE PROMISE OF HOMEOPATHY*

"*Sane Asylums* gives us an illuminating look into a time when visionary doctors treated mental illness with care, compassion, and gentle, effective homeopathic remedies. It is an important historical addition that will enlighten therapists as well as anyone interested in improving the treatment of those with severe mental illness. One can only hope that this history becomes better known so that all effective treatments, such as homeopathy, will flourish."

JANE TARA CICCHETTI, CCH, AUTHOR OF
*DREAMS, SYMBOLS, AND HOMEOPATHY*

"*Sane Asylums* is a book that makes you want to travel back in time and go to 1875–1925 when mental asylums in the United States offered humane living conditions, compassionate care, sports therapy, and homeopathic remedies to thousands of people with mental illness and obtained successful cures. *Sane Asylums* shows what was possible back then and what can be achieved today if the homeopathic approach to mental illness is made available again and we, as a society, learn to invest in sanity."

VATSALA SPERLING, PH.D., P.D.HOM, CCH, R.S.HOM,
CLASSICAL HOMEOPATH AND AUTHOR OF *THE AYURVEDIC RESET DIET*

"Highly recommended. *Sane Asylums* is an engaging, well-researched, and very much needed historical perspective on the role of homeopathy in the evolution of medicine in the United States. Rather than the 'scrubbed' historical version we are accustomed to finding in our history books, *Sane Asylums* sheds new light on homeopathy's relevance for mental health care, medicine, nursing, and politics today. Well worth the read!"

ANN MCKAY, RN-BC, CCH, HWNC-BC, HOMEOPATH

"In an insane world, what better than to challenge our collective cognitive dissonance around psychiatry? Homeopathy is biological intelligence and inheritance. Seems we knew this once upon a time. 'Mad' props to Jerry Kantor for uncovering beautiful, forgotten, misunderstood, and disavowed parts of our medical history."

LOUISE KUO, HEALTH FREEDOM ACTIVIST
AND AUTHOR OF *VACCINE EPIDEMIC*

"Do you like history, homeopathic history? Well then, you're sure to appreciate Jerry Kantor's inspiring scholarship in this psychological thriller. And what's most unsettling is that it's all true!"

JAY YASGUR, AUTHOR OF *YASGUR'S HOMEOPATHIC DICTIONARY
AND HOLISTIC HEALTH REFERENCE*

# SANE ASYLUMS

The Success of Homeopathy
before Psychiatry
Lost Its Mind

## JERRY M. KANTOR

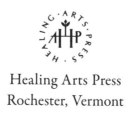

Healing Arts Press
Rochester, Vermont

Healing Arts Press
One Park Street
Rochester, Vermont 05767
www.HealingArtsPress.com

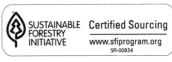

Text stock is SFI certified

Healing Arts Press is a division of Inner Traditions International

*Note to the reader: This book is intended as an informational guide. The remedies, approaches, and techniques described herein are meant to supplement, and not to be a substitute for, professional medical care or treatment. They should not be used to treat a serious ailment without prior consultation with a qualified health care professional.*

Cataloging-in-Publication Data for this title is available from the Library of Congress

ISBN 978-1-64411-408-7 (print)
ISBN 978-1-64411-409-4 (ebook)

Printed and bound in the United States by Lake Book Manufacturing, Inc. The text stock is SFI certified. The Sustainable Forestry Initiative® program promotes sustainable forest management.

10  9  8  7  6  5  4  3  2  1

Text design and layout by Virginia Scott Bowman
This book was typeset in Garamond Premier Pro with Bembo and Gill Sans used as display typefaces

To send correspondence to the author of this book, mail a first-class letter to the author c/o Inner Traditions • Bear & Company, One Park Street, Rochester, VT 05767, and we will forward the communication, or contact the author directly at **vitalforcehealthcare.com**.

*Dedicated to the memory of Selden H. Talcott*

# Contents

# Foreword

## By Eric Leskowitz, M.D.

Homeopathy, psychiatry, baseball, and synchronicity: these are the four factors that led me to write the foreword to this fascinating book.

Let's start with the synchronicity. Exactly two hours before being invited by Jerry Kantor to write this foreword, a friend suggested that I read an essay on the website Mad in America about a support group for people who hear voices but don't use psych meds. It turned out that the website's founder, an anti-psychiatry journalist I'd never heard of, is a primary source and major influence in *Sane Asylums*. This sign was impossible to ignore, even if my logical mind couldn't explain how synchronicity works. Ironically, that is the same issue facing homeopaths like Jerry Kantor, because mainstream medicine doesn't know how homeopathy works and thus finds it easy to dismiss.

I'm a holistic licensed psychiatrist now, but throughout my medical school and psychiatric training, the ultimate put-down to any new approach to therapy was to compare it to the modus operandi of homeopathy—titration: "How could it possibly work? There aren't even any molecules of the original substance left!" Even though my clinical practice generally focuses on mind/body approaches such as meditation and hypnosis (and another difficult-to-explain therapy—energy healing), I had never warmed to homeopathy. So it was ironic when some of my colleagues at Spaulding Rehabilitation Hospital in Boston were awarded one of the first pilot grants from the National Institutes of Health (NIH) in the area of alternative medicine (as it was called then), to study the efficacy of homeopathic treatments for mild traumatic brain injury.

This was in 1992, when the NIH's total research budget for alternative medicine was $300,000 (it's now $150 million) and Spaulding was not yet academically affiliated with Harvard Medical School. That small grant ($30,000) actually represented the first time we'd received any federal funding for research, and although it's only a pittance compared to Spaulding's current research budget, it was a source of immense pride for our hospital director. Except for one minor detail . . .

How was he going to brag about his NIH grant when its focus was a technique that he, and the rest of the Boston medical community, believed was quackery, plain and simple? It was my first chance to learn about homeopathy, because I served on the study's institutional review board and I saw the unrealistic constraints that had to be followed (for example, being limited to prescribing, from the vast pharmacopoeia of homeopathy, one of only ten total remedies that had been preapproved for the study, rather than the remedy that best matched the patient's symptoms). Yet despite this catch-22, the project unfolded smoothly and produced positive results.

The project's principal investigator was a psychiatrist who escaped these constraints by leaving academia and going into private practice. But times are changing, and Mr. Kantor's book helps us to appreciate just how big the changes have been, by first showing where the pendulum was almost 150 years ago, during homeopathy's heyday before psychiatry's post-WWII swing back to the world of medications and symptom suppression. Hopefully his book will help with the growing reacceptance of the healing modality of homeopathy, as well as the rebalancing of psychiatry.

I've gotten to know Jerry Kantor over my past thirty years as a holistic medicine pioneer in Boston. It's an academic hub that's not at all receptive to novel approaches, so I appreciate how significant it is that, in addition to being a homeopath, Jerry was the first acupuncturist (he's dually trained) to be granted a faculty position at Harvard Medical School's Department of Anaesthesiology. That says a lot about how well respected he is. And—full disclosure—years ago I saw him for a personal health consultation. I've forgotten the symptom being addressed, but I still remember that he found an uncannily precise constitutional remedy for me based on some seemingly random and irrelevant personality quirks. It seems there was method to his madness, and it worked, even if we didn't know how.

That not-knowing is a key point in homeopathy: How does it work? We certainly use other treatments that have mechanisms we don't understand; general anesthesia is a common one.* Kantor addresses this objection head-on by giving an elegant presentation of "nanoparticle cross-adaptation." I was intrigued to learn that the model he invoked was a key part of the defense testimony in a landmark lawsuit filed against a homeopathic product manufacturer in 2015; scientifically inclined readers may enjoy appendix 2, which includes a concise summary of this research that was powerful enough to convince the court to dismiss all charges against the manufacturer, including the requested $250 million in damages.

In another appendix, Kantor addresses the cross-cultural issues raised by the topic of mental illness itself, since what is perceived as insanity in one culture may be a valued behavior in another. His extensive Compendium of Madness Perspectives offers a range of interpretations from around the world, material that could form the basis for an entire separate book, ranging from Buddhism's "crazy wisdom" and Christianity's "dark night of the soul," to "melancholia," "blood lust," and "monomania." In addition to these appendices, Kantor includes prints and photos of a number of so-called mental hospitals that are in the American Institute of Homeopathy's archives. The illustrations are a highlight of the book, with naturalistic settings that are in stark contrast to the dehumanizing, institutionalized style of modern psychiatric hospitals.

There are also some vintage and initially puzzling portrait photos of baseball teams from the 1870s and '80s. It turns out that one of the

---

*Against the argument that anesthesia simply requires interruption of nerve conduction, many numbing substances don't allow surgical-depth anesthesia—that is, pain blockage that can withstand normally painful incisions. Something different goes on with anesthetics (ether, laughing gas, halothane) compared to Oxycontin or Valium, and it's a mystery why Substance A can be used for surgery while Substance B cannot. Inspection of the chemical compound's structure does not help us predict which substance will work.

early homeopathic asylums discovered that their patients loved to watch the staff play baseball and so fielded its own amateur baseball team as a way to build morale and team spirit. The team was good enough to beat all amateur challengers and even played exhibition matches against a professional team. Kantor doesn't say whether they took any homeopathic remedies as performance enhancers, but if these remedies were used in sports today, they would have the benefit of being undetectable to drug testing.

In addition to five appendices there are numerous useful references and a convenient list of online resources that the reader will appreciate. These dozens of pages of material are just tasty side dishes to the main course, the twelve chapters that comprise the core of the book. They are diverse and thorough, beginning with an overview of the history of homeopathy and the era of moral care, and highlighting how Dr. Samuel Hahnemann developed his approach as a counter to the harsh medical treatments of the late eighteenth century (blood-letting, leeching, purging, and so on). His view that symptoms represent the body's natural defenses rather than the disease itself was in major disagreement with prevailing medical standards, which have often viewed symptoms as the enemy to be defeated or suppressed. Homeopathy, in contrast, works to strengthen the body so it can heal itself and cast off the symptoms. As word of Hahnemann's clinical successes spread through Europe and then America, homeopathic clinics were established based on his system, and eventually hospitals were built. Many American cities still have hospitals named after Hahnemann, though they no longer officially practice homeopathy and generally underplay their connection to this school of therapeutics.

One little known and particularly interesting story concerning the acceptance of homeopathy is the role it played in helping Mary Todd Lincoln, widow of our sixteenth president, to recover from the emotional shock of her husband's assassination. Kantor's detective work uncovered connections that had not previously been addressed in the literature on homeopathy or in American history, yet another example of the suppression of information that doesn't support our dominant medical narrative. His recounting of "The Madness of Mary Todd

Lincoln" (chapter 4) deserves to be widely read, and hopefully this book will be the vehicle for bringing such important information to a wider audience.

A guiding light in American homeopathy, Selden Talcott, M.D.—wryly described by Kantor as "perhaps the greatest psychiatrist this country has ever (not) known"—is the focus of chapters 5 and 6, the latter describing the utopian agenda of his Middletown State Homeopathic Hospital of New York State. This approach included occupational therapy, a sanctuary, and medical research into individualized treatments for its residents. Treatment approaches included "kindness and gentle discipline," massage, bed rest, dietetics, exercise, amusement, and "moral hygiene," described as "soul encouragement from the strong to the weak." These approaches are described in detail and leave a strong impression of care for the mentally ill that is driven by humane concerns rather than financial ones.

Sample diagnoses and treatment plans from that era are interspersed in these chapters, along with other historical nuggets that are on par with the revelation (to me, at least) that one of the three Menninger doctors who founded their Houston, Texas, psychiatric clinic was a homeopath, as was the founder of Boston University Medical School's nationally respected Solomon Carter Fuller Mental Health Center.

Another timely piece of history relates not to mental health but to the treatment of flu epidemics. Kantor presents reporting that shows the Spanish Flu of 1918 was rapidly and effectively treated by homeopaths, while the standard medical treatment of that era—including unsafe mega-doses of the new wonder drug aspirin—might have caused conflicting symptoms and confusion, thus contributing to the devastating spread of the disease.

His final chapter, "Investing in Sanity," is a reasoned plea to use less expensive, less dangerous, and more humane methods in our treatment of the psychiatrically impaired. It would be difficult to argue with that goal.

In summary, I highly recommend *Sane Asylums* to anyone interested in homeopathy, the history (and future) of medicine, alternative views of health and illness, and America's national pastime of baseball.

We have a lot to learn from history, and Kantor's book is an elegant teacher and guide.

ERIC LESKOWITZ, M.D., the founder of EnergyMedicine101.com, is a board-certified psychiatrist with the Pain Management Program at Spaulding Rehabilitation Hospital in Boston, where he directs the hospital's Integrative Medicine Task Force. He was a faculty member of the Department of Psychiatry of Harvard Medical School for twenty years, has organized several conferences on the topic of complementary and alternative medicine in rehabilitation, and has written and lectured widely on the field of energy medicine.

# Preface

This book is intended for a wide range of readers: those disillusioned with modern psychopharmacology, wondering if there is a better way; and those seeking to bring forward evidence for the effectiveness of homeopathy. It will also resonate with readers who have diverse interests such as the psychological benefits of baseball or the mystery of Mary Todd Lincoln's illness. The scope of this book includes the following:

- Presents a vision of mental health care for the future predicated on a model that flourished for half a century and worked more effectively than anything we are doing now. This model entailed humane, compassionate care and fulfilling activities within a bucolic setting, along with the use of homeopathics, and still outperforms mainstream medicine for mental health in a multitude of instances.
- Excavates a closeted history, that of homeopathic mental hospitals, their doctors, and their nurses from the post–Civil War era into the 1930s. This exploration confers overdue appreciation for the work of physicians Selden Talcott and his brilliant colleague Clara Barrus at the inspired Middletown State Homeopathic Hospital.
- Brings a practitioner's eye to bear on homeopathy's advent into neuropsychiatry with an introduction to public health pioneer Samuel Hahnemann, founder of the system of therapeutics known as homeopathy, including the principles he espoused and the medicines he prescribed. Hahnemann's documented cure of

an Austrian nobleman's insanity deserves special credit.

■ Solves the mystery of Abraham Lincoln's widow, Mary Todd Lincoln, and her descent into madness following the loss of her husband and two sons amid scurrilous political rumors. I present new and compelling evidence that she recovered from mental illness through homeopathy and evidence that Abraham Lincoln himself was a lifelong user of homeopathic medicine.

■ Spreads the word that safe and effective redress of mental illness has long been at hand. Author Robert Whitaker's books *Anatomy of an Epidemic: Magic Bullets, Psychiatric Drugs, and the Astonishing Rise of Mental Illness in America*; *Mad in America: Bad Science, Bad Medicine, and the Enduring Mistreatment of the Mentally Ill*; and *Psychiatry under the Influence: Institutional Corruption, Social Injury, and Prescriptions for Reform* damn psychopharmacology and demand a response. Disclosure of the homeopathic record and unprejudiced access to homeopathy's science and medicines can inform that response. It is suggested that aligning with homeopathy would galvanize the Mad in America and anti-psychiatry movements.

■ Supports Dr. Thomas Szasz, whose 1961 book, *The Myth of Mental Illness: Foundations of a Theory of Personal Conduct,* presents his doubts concerning psychiatry's legitimacy. In an essay summarizing his position Szasz states, "Psychiatry, I submit, is very much more intimately tied to problems of ethics than is medicine. I use the word 'psychiatry' here to refer to that contemporary discipline which is concerned with *problems in living* (and not with diseases of the brain, which are problems for neurology)."[1] Though himself a respected psychiatrist, Szasz's argument failed to gain traction. Meanwhile, Syracuse University Medical School, where Szasz taught for several decades, has in his absence—all while collecting royalties on his books—committed itself to teaching the very psychopharmacology that Dr. Szasz dismissed as rubbish. Substantiating his position, a 2019 study published in *Psychiatry Research* concluded that psychiatric diagnoses are "scientifically meaningless" as tools to explain discrete mental health disorders, revealing little about individual experience and complex causes.

- Contextualizes homeopathy's decline and explains why the Middletown State Homeopathic Hospital and its satellites nose-dived from the 1930s on, the asylums eventually growing indistinguishable from other dismally operated psychiatric facilities. Now, rather than commemorating an inspiring era of medical healing, internet images of dilapidated buildings and haunted destinations lure Halloween thrill-seekers.[2] As if the torturous treatments that for so long were visited upon the mentally ill had anything to do with homeopathy, the designation "Homeopathic" mockingly adorns at least one ruined facility's front gates. As an antidote to this I am pleased to acquaint the reader with this history and share a sampling of the 1916 American Institute of Homeopathy's 199 images documenting more than one hundred homeopathic hospitals and sanatoriums as they appeared in their prime.
- Explores the rationale for baseball therapy and showcases Middletown Hospital's celebrated baseball team, the Asylums.
- Provides a global compendium of perspectives concerning madness.
- Introduces Dr. Iris Bell's validation and recasting of homeopathy as nanomedicine.

Homeopathic products induce a holistic response. That does not mean every holistic product or all gentle-acting medicines are homeopathic. Within the limited selection of natural foods and supplement outlets, homeopathics must often share shelf space with herbs, nutritional supplements, and other non-drug commodities whose modes of action are entirely non-homeopathic. By providing context to homeopathy's rich heritage, this text hopes to alleviate widespread confusion concerning homeopathic medicines.

⊕

My thanks go out to Richard Grossinger and Dana Ullman for their championing of this book; Burke Lennihan for her sharp eyes and sage advice; Bob Mayer for allowing access to his wonderful baseball archive; Francis Treuherz and Robert Juette for sharing their intimate knowledge of homeopathy's origins; Judi Calvert for her unstinting efforts to supply me with resources; Jhuma Biswas for being my sounding board; Norman Waksler for moral support; and Theo Epstein for his homeopathic revamping of the Boston Red Sox roster that in 2004 ended the curse of the Bambino.

A hand to the heart for Emily Coyne, the little girl whose gift of an inscrolled wish that I write another book, placed in a decorated miniature vial, inspired me. Appreciation and gratitude go out to Dr. Eric Leskowitz for his splendid foreword; my marvelous editor Jamaica Burns Griffin; and my wife, Hannah, for her many clear-eyed suggestions and constant support.

----------------------------------------

# The Dead Sea Scrolls of Homeopathy and Psychiatry

*All censorships exist to prevent anyone from challenging current conceptions and existing institutions. All progress is initiated by challenging current conceptions, and executed by supplanting existing institutions. Consequently, the first condition of progress is the removal of censorship.*

GEORGE BERNARD SHAW,
*MRS. WARREN'S PROFESSION*

The Dead Sea Scrolls, ancient religious texts rediscovered in 1947 in a remote cave, are estimated by scholars to date from the last three centuries BCE and the first century CE. The documents referred to in this text date back only a few centuries but are quite powerful in what they reveal about America's treatment of the mentally ill. Rather than emerging as a trove of documents, the revelations have unfolded through painstaking and persistent research.

## A ROAD NOT TAKEN

*Sane Asylums* is a century and a half retrospective to a Camelot of health care, a time when an effective and utopian approach to mental illness prevailed. Knowledge of this flourishing homeopathic era and its advanced methods remains inconvenient to the economic interests of psychopharmacology. *Sane Asylums'* aim is to examine this past history so that a new path forward in the care and treatment of the mentally ill can be imagined.

Has psychiatry gone astray? It appears so, with corporate greed as the primary cause. Despite what some consider state-of-the art psychiatric treatment, rather than declining the number of identified disabled mentally ill has tripled in this country in the past twenty years. Ever more patients with intractable and increasingly dire diagnoses requiring medication continue to appear. In turn, the need to counter the side effects of these same medications has escalated.

As Robert Whitaker shows in *Anatomy of an Epidemic,* simply not using psychiatric medication enables the poorest and least developed countries in the world to consistently outperform the United States across all measures with regard to short- and long-term schizophrenia outcomes. Need one doubt that a craving for market expansion propels the skyrocketing census of depressed and bipolar individuals? Or that this is the reason why healthy youngsters are suddenly earmarked for psychopharmacology's tender mercies?

Psychiatry need not have gone down this road. In fact, for a quarter of a century, throughout much of the United States alternate and well-traveled routes for humane and effective psychiatric care existed. Whether mentally or physically ill, people flocked to homeopaths because these physicians *listened to,* rather than condescended to, their patients. Whereas conventional physicians of that era prescribed on the basis of often dubious biological suppositions directing them to ply a patient with toxic mercury or bleed them repeatedly, their homeopathic counterparts prescribed gentle medicines attuned to the stresses and influences responsible for their patient's symptoms. Which doctor would you have chosen?

Are the utopian homeopathic asylums of the turn of the nineteenth century a myth? One might think so based on a dearth of their mention in contemporary historical medical literature. Readers of influential texts such as *Madness: An American History of Mental Illness and Its Treatment* will puzzle over why author Mary de Young's chapter on asylums declines to mention homeopathy's numerous mental hospitals. The omission fosters a preferred reality in which the hospitals never existed. In fact, many American hospitals and medical schools had homeopathic founders and boasted countless homeopathically directed activities, mention of which has been scrubbed from most history.

I consider the information *Sane Asylums* presents to be a corollary to the Dead Sea Scrolls, which illuminated a wide spectrum of ancient beliefs and practices; this information, however, is only a few centuries old, as opposed to two thousand years. It was not smuggled from the caves of Qumran but secreted in wilted letters and journals; the minutes of physician organizations; bygone texts; rare offerings of publishers Forgotten Books, Kissinger Publishing L.L.C., and the Wentworth Press; and the University of Michigan Library's digitalization of dusty archives. Still, the material will enlighten.

Medical historians accustomed to hailing French physician Philippe Pinel as the first doctor to replace brutal care of the mentally ill with psychologically oriented humanitarian (or what Pinel called "moral") care will have to reconsider. What I am terming the "Dead Sea Scrolls of homeopathy" reveal that these contemporaries must share credit. Pinel made human changes in treatment, but it was Samuel Hahnemann who pioneered homeopathic remediation in an asylum in Georgenthal, Germany, in 1792.

Online searchers, unaware that shills for the pharmacology industry have commandeered the Wikipedia homeopathy page, take the website's disparaging account as gospel truth.[1] Shown otherwise they will scratch their heads. So too might visitors to the website of the American Medical Association (AMA), where an exalted account of the organization's origins is given the lie by economist Dale Steinreich's sordid revelation: "AMA's initial drive to increase physician incomes was motivated by increasing competition from homeopaths. . . . In the year before AMA's founding, the *New York Journal of Medicine* stated that competition with homeopathy caused 'a large pecuniary loss' to allopaths."[2] And in 1872, one allopath embroiled in the controversy at the University of Michigan, where a professorship in homeopathy had been established since 1855, argued that the university was "throwing discouragements in the path of the graduates in scientific medicine and rendering the struggle for existence more arduous and unremunerative."[3]

## FURTHER REVELATIONS

Homeopathy's popularity in the nineteenth and early twentieth century is evident from its celebrated advocates, including luminaries William James, Henry Wadsworth Longfellow, Nathanial Hawthorne, Harriet Beecher Stowe, Daniel Webster, William Seward, Horace Greeley, Louisa May Alcott, and journalist William Cullen Bryant (who served for a time as president of the Homeopathic Medical Society of the State of New York).[4]

There have been more than one hundred homeopathic hospitals and twenty-two homeopathic medical schools in the United States. These included forerunners of Drexel University College of Medicine (representing the legacies of two historic medical schools, Hahnemann Medical College and the Women's Medical College of Pennsylvania), Boston University, Stanford University, New York Medical College, University of Michigan, and more than a thousand homeopathic pharmacies.

## HOMEOPATHY AMID PANDEMICS

Amid today's Covid-19 pandemic, historian Julian Winston's disclosures concerning homeopathy's effectiveness during other major epidemics are relevant. From his introduction to "Influenza–1918: Homeopathy to the Rescue" article published in 1998:

> It was called "the Great White Plague." It is hard to imagine the devastation caused by the flu epidemic of 1918–19. People who lived through it reported that someone who was up and well in the morning could be dead by evening.

Winston goes on to quote the following testimonials compiled by Dean W. A. Pearson of Philadelphia and included in a 1920 article by W. A. Dewey, M.D., titled "Homeopathy in Influenza—A Chorus of Fifty in Harmony," which appeared in the *Journal of the American Institute of Homeopathy*. Pearson recorded 26,795 cases of influenza treated by homeopathic physicians with a mortality of 1.05 percent, while the average mainstream medicine mortality was 30 percent.

In the transport service I had 81 cases on the way over. All recovered and were landed. Every man received homeopathic treatment. One [non-homeopathic] ship lost 31 on the way.

—H. A. ROBERTS, M.D., DERBY, CONNECTICUT

In a plant of 8,000 workers we had only one death. The patients were not drugged to death. Gelsemium was practically the only remedy used. We used no aspirin and no vaccines.

—FRANK WIELAND, M.D., CHICAGO

I did not lose a single case of influenza; my death rate in the pneumonias was 2.1%. The salicylates, including aspirin and quinine, were almost the sole standbys of the old school and it was a common thing to hear them speaking of losing 60% of their pneumonias.

—DUDLEY A. WILLIAMS, M.D., PROVIDENCE, RHODE ISLAND

Fifteen hundred cases were reported at the Homeopathic Medical Society of the District of Columbia with but fifteen deaths. Recoveries in the National Homeopathic Hospital were 100%.

—E. F. SAPPINGTON, M.D., PHILADELPHIA

I have treated 1,000 cases of influenza. I have the records to show my work. I have no losses. Please give all credit to homeopathy!

—T. A. MCCANN, M.D., DAYTON, OHIO

One physician in a Pittsburgh hospital asked a nurse if she knew anything better than what he was doing, because he was losing many cases. "Yes, Doctor, stop aspirin and go down to a homeopathic pharmacy, and get homeopathic remedies." The doctor replied: "But that is homeopathy." "I know it, but the homeopathic doctors for whom I have nursed have not lost a single case."

—W. F. EDMUNDSON, M.D., PITTSBURGH

*Three hundred and fifty cases and lost one, a neglected pneumonia that came to me after she had taken one hundred grains of aspirin in twenty-four hours.*

—CORA SMITH KING, M.D., WASHINGTON, D.C.

*I had a package handed to me containing 1,000 aspirin tablets, which was 994 too many. I think I gave about a half dozen. I almost invariably gave Gelsemium and Bryonia. I hardly ever lost a case if I got there first, unless the patient had been sent to a drug store and bought aspirin, in which event I was likely to have a case of pneumonia on my hands.*

—J. P. HUFF, M.D., OLIVE BRANCH, KENTUCKY

In reading the accounts of the epidemic it seems that most of the deaths were caused by a virulent pneumonia that was especially devastating to those who depressed their systems with analgesics, the most common being aspirin.[5]

## THE MOTHER CHURCH: MIDDLETOWN, NEW YORK, HOMEOPATHIC HOSPITAL

After opening its doors in 1874, New York's Middletown State Homeopathic Hospital flourished for twenty-five years. Its third superintendent, Selden Talcott, planned and oversaw a treatment regime marrying Quaker physician Thomas Kirkbride's moral treatment principles of compassion and respect to scientific medicine. Talcott's methods inspired ardent disciples and similarly enlightened asylums across the country. The many failings of contemporary psychiatry and the omission of homeopathy's successes from historical accounts entreat reconsideration—if not celebration—of Talcott's work and legacy.

Psychiatry since 1875 has regressed. Its feckless lack of concern for the addictiveness of its drugs abetted the heedless prescribing responsible for the opioid crisis. Modern psychiatry also has limited tools for countering symptoms of present-day autism and often includes broadly prescribed psychoactive drugs or anticonvulsants with potentially risky side effects; whereas homeopathy is able to target a specific remedy for each case that can address all the symptoms. According to the findings of Robert Whitaker, the field has also midwifed a host of previously nonexistent psychiatric ailments, all while spurring exponential growth of the mentally ill. He shows how widespread use of lobotomies in the 1920s and '30s gave way in the 1950s to electroshock and a wave of new drugs.[6]

Whitaker explodes a myth: that the advent of Thorazine eliminated the need for mental asylums (changes in institutional reimbursement caused that), and by referencing the profession's own studies documents the iatrogenic harm caused by psychopharmacology: rampant mania, psychosis, hallucination, depersonalization, suicidal ideation, heart attack, stroke, and sudden death. He documents how schizophrenics in the United States currently fare worse than patients in the world's poorest and least developed countries, that modern treatments for the severely mentally ill recycle failed toxic and suppressive approaches, and that society's delusion about their efficacy is continually stoked by profiteering interests. Damningly, he reveals how while refusing to disclose dangerous side effects to patients, pharmaceutical companies in the 1980s and '90s rigged their studies so that new antipsychotic medications could appear more effective than old ones.

A 2019 study published in *Psychiatry Research* concluded, "A pragmatic approach to psychiatric assessment, allowing for recognition of individual experience, may therefore be a more effective way of understanding distress than maintaining commitment to a *disingenuous categorical system*"[7] (italics mine).

By contrast, Middletown State Homeopathic Hospital for the insane was unparalleled, a virtually self-sufficient New York utopia. Funded by the state, it was a thoughtfully designed complex of forty-seven buildings situated on bucolic grounds with more than two thousand beds. Its patients gardened, played and listened to music, practiced artistry, exercised, received occupational therapy, and participated in and watched baseball games. Compared with the barbaric physical restraints and moralistically inspired torments on tap within other asylums of the time, Middletown was a hospital where a nutritious diet, compassionate care, and sophisticated side effect–free homeopathic prescriptions produced cures for a range of ills. Among these were supposedly intractable conditions such as dementia praecox (currently thought to be an amalgam of schizophrenia and encephalitis lethargica).

Selden Talcott was arguably the greatest psychiatrist America has (not) known. The physician Clara Barrus, who supervised the nurses, was a brilliant holistic thinker. The fruits of their labors and those of their disciples command a second look. In addition to amending the historical record, *Sane Asylums* presents homeopathy's theory, scientific basis, and an account of its eclipse. Middletown's treatments and medicines (most of which homeopaths use to this day) are brought to life. It is hoped that *Sane Asylums* will spur debate about the mentally ill and the critical role homeopathy can play in their care.

## CONCERNING PARLANCE

Though *Sane Asylums* reinstates an earlier era, words then commonly in use, such as *insanity, madness, lunatic,* and *imbecility,* offend the modern ear. *Alcoholism* is more familiar than *inebriation.* Whenever possible I use modern language and more respectful terms to refer to the mentally ill. When period authenticity requires recourse to more archaic usage, an explanation will be offered.

Despite frequent rebranding with names such as lunatic asylum, insane asylum, state hospital, mental institution, mental hospital, psychiatric hospital, psychiatric campus, and the like, the term *asylum* has retained its original meaning as a place proffering refuge and assistance, and so it will be our principal term of reference.

### A Word about Spelling

Just as language and branding have evolved, so too has spelling: homoeopathy has been simplified to homeopathy; anaesthesiology is now known as anesthesiology; and many European names and words have lost their accent marks. Throughout this book you'll find spelling variations as we endeavor to remain true to our source material yet bow to contemporary preferred usage.

# 1

## Who Are the Mad and Where Shall They Dwell?

*We have deceived ourselves that having a home and being mentally healthy are our natural conditions, and that we become homeless or mentally ill as a result of "losing" our homes or our minds. The opposite is the case. We are born without a home and without reason, and have to exert ourselves and are fortunate if we succeed in building a secure home and a sound mind. . . . the terms "home" and "mental health" refer to complex, personal traits-as-possessions, which must be acquired, cultivated, and maintained by ceaseless effort.*

THOMAS SZASZ, *CRUEL COMPASSION: PSYCHIATRIC CONTROL OF SOCIETY'S UNWANTED*

To "Who are the mad and where shall they dwell?" we can append, "And how long are they permitted to dwell there?" Or, given the amount of mental illness found among the homeless today, is it permissible for them to dwell anywhere at all?

### HOPE FOR THE MENTALLY ILL

*Sane Asylums* illuminates a half century, roughly 1875 to 1925, when homeopathically directed hospitals for the mentally ill in America proliferated, thrived, and conducted themselves in a respectful, compassionate, and nurturing manner toward their residents. Given their visionary, often self-sustaining design, innovations, and documented success with a challenging population, to speak of such asylums as enlightened is no exaggeration.

Perspectives concerning mental illness and behavior toward the mentally ill comprise a landscape with ever-shifting economic, sociological, psychological, and medical features. Prior to engaging with the asylums we inquire, "Who are the mad who voluntarily or involuntarily dwell there?" Most importantly, "Who are the mad?" is about threat, power, and privilege. It is vexing to consider these questions: Shall the mad dwell among us or apart from us? Under what means of restraint shall they dwell? For how long and in what settings should they be restrained? Here is how psychiatrist Thomas Szasz, who questioned the legitimacy of his field, put it:

> For millennia the dialectic of vilification and deification, and, more generally, of invalidation and validation—excluding the individual from the group as an evil outsider or including him in it as a member in good standing—was cast in the imagery and rhetoric of magic and religion. . . . With the decline of the religious worldview and the ascent of the scientific method during the Renaissance and the Enlightenment, the religious rhetoric of validation and invalidation was gradually replaced by the scientific. One of the most dramatic results of this transformation is the lexicon of psychiatric diagnoses functioning as a powerful, but largely unacknowledged, rhetoric of rejection and stigmatization.[1]

Such questions entreat consideration of social, economic, religious, and political context. For Selden Talcott and his disciples, insanity was a medical and homeopathic issue. Doctors too must shift perspective. How to best treat the mentally ill is never a settled matter.

## SEVEN CATEGORIES

The perception of mental illness in pre-psychopharmaceutical times differed from today, when proliferating iatrogenic conditions are accepted as both commonplace and normal. To bridge the gap between disparate eras, seven perspective-based categories of mental illness are offered. The appendices offer an elaboration of this breakdown with a variety of perspectives distilled from an array of cultures and contexts.

### *The Mentally Ill as Beasts*

Within Europe, rationalism was understood as an appeal to human reason as a means of acquiring knowledge. A chief proponent was René Descartes (1596–1650), a mathematician who espoused the belief that the knowledge of eternal truths could be attained by reason alone and without recourse to experience. Philosopher Benedict Spinoza and philosopher/mathematician Gottfried Wilhelm Leibniz both promoted this ideal with regard to scientific knowledge. Within Britain the empirically oriented pre-Enlightenment branch of rationalism, which emphasized the role of sensory experience as opposed to reasoning in acquiring knowledge, was taught by philosophers George Berkeley, John Locke, and David Hume.

If—as the sages of the eighteenth and nineteenth century claimed— man is the rational animal, then what is to be made of the mad, who have lost their reason? The unavoidable answer was that they would thus be nothing other than beasts and should be treated as such. This understanding justified barbaric interventions such as the following: confinement in a small room or cell, chaining to a post, beatings intended to "domesticate" them, frightening them, submerging them in ice water, forcing them to vomit, applying caustic substances to their skin to draw out the ill humors, and fixing them with an intense gaze, all of which were deemed to have the salutary effect of keeping the mad tractable.

When the mad are viewed as beasts they are prone to being jailed or compelled to reside in the worst of asylums, such as the inhumane Bedlam (Bethlem) in London, founded in 1247. It was relocated in

1930 to Beckenham, Kent, where it still functions today, albeit in a more humane iteration.

## The Mentally Ill as Possessed

The hallucinating member of a religious community in almost any age can be viewed as being distracted from piety by a devilish or evil spirit. Within Puritan New England the thin line between distraction and wickedness due to possession was momentous. Hanging in the balance was Puritan minister Cotton Mather's determination: the distracted Pilgrim in question was to be either remanded to intense Bible study in the home or subjected to torture and execution.

Alternatively, the treatment of madness via ritual exorcism is widespread throughout clerical settings of every religion and shamanic tradition. The procedures can involve drumming, prayer, incantation, dancing, trance, visions, illusions of light, ingesting herbs, interacting with snakes, receiving massage, and sleep deprivation.

Within the asylum setting, investment in madness due to possession has inspired trephination (piercing the skull with a surgical instrument), salutary electrocution (a cruder forerunner of electroconvulsive therapy), and waterboarding in the hope that a near-death experience proves purgative. When the mad are viewed as possessed, they are more likely to be maintained and dealt with within their communal or tribal setting.

## The Mentally Ill as Sinners

Closely aligned with the notion of demonic possession is the belief taught in the Bible that madness is punishment for sinful behavior. Two examples:

> "The Lord will smite you with madness, blindness, and bewilderment of heart." (Deut. 28:27–29)
> "God will send upon them a deluding influence [delusion] so that they will believe what is false." (2 Thess. 2:11)

The sinner stands by powerless to resist madness generated by God's wrath. On the other hand, prior to being smitten with madness his freedom of choice would have invited him to rein in his greed, lust, desire for drink, impulse to gamble, outsized social or political ambitions, or desire to transgress God's will. Immersion in prayer, modesty, piety, philanthropy, fasting, sexual restraint, and an orientation toward humility are proactive measures fending off madness.

So that God's curse can perhaps be lifted, the belief goes, we must pray for those afflicted by madness. If the clerical word *sinning* is replaced with the secular term *injudicious choice,* alternative measures can ensue. Those whose weakness of will has delivered them into ruin and madness can be offered not just prayers but also respectful moral redirection, an environment devoid of temptation, and realizable incentives to stability. Where the mad are viewed as sinners they become the target of browbeating and religiously based efforts at reform, such as evangelism within clerical settings—churches, synagogues, and tent ministries. See also *dybbuk* in appendix 1.

### The Mentally Ill as Diseased
### (Poisoned, Brain Injured, Hereditarily Impaired)
Again, Dr. Thomas Szasz states:

Mental illness, of course, is not literally a "thing"—or physical object—and hence it can "exist" only in the same sort of way in which other theoretical concepts exist. Yet, familiar theories are in the habit of posing, sooner or later—at least to those who come to believe in them—as "objective truths" (or "facts").[2]

Historically many physical conditions have been misdiagnosed as psychological or neurological symptoms. The following conditions are empirically confirmable via medical technologies, such as brain scanning, biopsy, and blood testing:

- Traumatic brain injury, which can cause personality changes, emotional lability (mood swings), depression and sense of loss, anxiety, spasticity, apraxia (a motor speech disorder), frustration, and anger. Also post-traumatic stress disorder (PTSD) and dementia as from multiple concussions resulting in chronic traumatic encephalopathy (CTE).

- Brain aneurysm: memory loss, confusion, loss of consciousness, diminished ability to concentrate.
- Anxiety disorders, which can atrophy regions of the brain (causes are not fully understood, according to the Mayo Clinic).[3]
- Ischemic or hemorrhagic stroke: slurred speech and confusion.
- Brain tumor: depression, irritability, amnesia.
- Depressive disorders.[4]
- Hypoxic injuries due to near-drowning, drug overdose, poisonings (such as carbon monoxide) leading to confusion. There may be brief jerks of the limbs (myoclonus) and seizures.
- Drug and alcohol addictions.
- Nervous system injuries as from exposure to heavy metals such as lead (cognitive loss), mercury (erethism, see appendix 1, "Compendium of Madness Perspectives"), alumina (confusion, loss of executive function).
- Epilepsy. According to the Mayo Clinic, epilepsy, a central nervous system disorder in which brain activity becomes abnormal, has no identifiable cause in half the people with the condition. Seizure conditions can vary greatly, ranging from vacant staring in absence seizures (previously known as petit mal seizures) to uncontrollable twitching, thrashing, and loss of consciousness in grand mal seizures.[5]

The following conditions when not directly attributable to pathology can be confirmed only by after-the-fact association with tissue abnormality found upon autopsy. Often suppositions are hyped to appear as legitimate by the public relations arms of the pharmaceutical industry.

- Depression following heart surgery (understood as the traditional Chinese medicine version of the heart as "ruler of all organs").
- Dementia. Loss of cognitive function and memory as a result of damage to or loss of nerve cells and their connections in the

brain. The most common cause of dementia is Alzheimer's disease, but there is a range of types of dementia.
- Psychopaths and sociopaths.

The following conditions have thus far proved elusive in terms of both diagnosis and physical ramifications, in both the living and the dead. (Not to mention the fact that due to the heterogeneous nature of categories within *The Diagnostic and Statistical Manual of Mental Disorders, DSM-5,* establishment of diagnoses in general is conceded to be problematic in psychiatry, as alluded to earlier.)

- Autism.
- Schizophrenia (unpersuasive neurotransmitter studies).
- Psychogenic (selective) mutism. An individual with this disorder is capable of speaking but ceases to speak. This disorder affects about 1 percent of young children.

Often appearing in emergency or urgent care settings, the following demographic resides within the community or in prisons or nursing homes and is subject to a virtually unlimited array of management approaches. These range from pharmaceutical dosing to acupuncture, homeopathy, chiropractic, psychotherapy, counseling, nutritional supplementation, and recovery and rehabilitation techniques.

## The Mentally Ill as Defective
Treatments included sterilization, marital prohibition, experimentation, genetic counseling, or even euthanasia. When viewed as such this demographic is found in concentration camps, euthanasia clinics, experimental or sterilization treatment settings, asylums, jails, and nursing homes.

## The Mentally Ill as Tortured Souls
## (Accursed, Guilt Ridden, Seriously Bereaved)
Dr. Szasz writes:

> Our adversaries are not demons, witches, fate, or mental illness. We have no enemy whom we can fight, exorcise, or dispel by "cure."

What we do have are problems in living—whether these be biologic, economic, political, or sociopsychological. My argument was limited to the proposition that mental illness is a myth, whose function it is to disguise and thus render more palatable the bitter pill of moral conflicts in human relations.[6]

Those viewed as belonging to the following category are targeted for religious or spiritually motivated efforts on behalf of redemption. They reside in the community but can be found in counseling, psychotherapy, cults, veteran support facilities, addiction recovery, and rehabilitation settings, as well as suicide prevention and PTSD clinics.

## The Mentally Ill as Troublemakers
Dr. Szasz notes:

> Although (mental illness) might have been a useful concept in the nineteenth century, today it is scientifically worthless and socially harmful. In non-psychiatric circles mental illness all too often is considered to be whatever psychiatrists say it is. The answer to the question, "Who is mentally ill?" thus becomes: Those who are confined in mental hospitals or who consult psychiatrists in their private offices.[7]

> In the animal kingdom the rule is that one must eat or be eaten; in the human kingdom, it is define or be defined.[8]

What human behavior has at some time or other not been deemed aberrant, therefore needful of restraint? In accordance with the standard that the mad oblige a societal response only when posing a risk to harming themselves or others, the readily abused troublemaker category is preeminent. Its demographic covers overenthusiastic scientists, criminals, cranks, misanthropes, mischief makers, punks, tough guys, bullies, and delinquents; personalities such as self-righteous, garrulous, silent, morbidly inclined, highly imaginative, excitable, capricious, passionate, irritating, vengeful, and nervous; liars, con artists, squanderers, social-change activists, dissidents, revolutionaries, pacifists, ecoterrorists, anarchists, and recluses; and the grief stricken, the restless or peripatetic, and the indolent.

The matter of perspective is highly relevant. Given the broad latitude within these perspectives, many may find themselves qualified as mad. Or conversely, which of us when encountering distasteful behavior or notions has never been drawn to lash out?

Common practice in the early nineteenth century included "warning out" and "passing on" of unwelcome persons, meaning loading them onto a cart and dropping them off in the next town. (See appendix 1, "warning out.") In contemporary times it is more likely to be a bus than a cart, but the practice is still a common way for cities to handle their "homeless problem."

In the twenty-first century the question persists: Do we prefer to reside near, among, or apart from our mentally ill? Where shall they dwell?

# 2

## The Dawn of Enlightened Mental Health Care

*Mistress, both man and master is possessed,*
*I know it by their pale and deadly looks.*
*They must be bound and laid in some dark room.*

WILLIAM SHAKESPEARE,
*THE COMEDY OF ERRORS*, ACT IV, SCENE 4

The late nineteenth century was awash with idealism, spiritualism, and philosophical big thinking. Mary Baker Eddy's Christian Science movement was founded in Boston in 1879. Her juggernaut religion proclaimed that Jesus Christ was chiefly a healer, and prayer was a direct avenue to medical cure. Philosophical movements flowering in the era included Utilitarianism, Marxism, Positivism, Pragmatism, Transcendentalism, Social Darwinism, and, via the writings of Kierkegaard and Nietzsche, antecedents of both psychoanalysis and existentialism. Not merely abstract, the mental fervor was a call to action feeding experimentation and upheaval within religious, social, economic, political, and medical milieus. Emblematic of the zeitgeist, Leo Tolstoy's magnificent novel *War and Peace,* noted for its psychological analysis and emphasis on family relationships within the context of incipient war, was published in 1869.

Amid this panoply of "isms," the cataclysmic grief and roiling madness of post–Civil War America, enlightened homeopathic asylums burst upon the scene. Primary catalysts were utopians searching for an ideal, self-sustaining community; moral care avatars such as the French psychiatrist Philippe Pinel and Quakers William Tuke and Thomas Kirkbride; and aficionados of family patronage care for the mentally ill in the Belgian city of Geel, where in 1852 oversight of the guardianship model was transferred from the Catholic Church to medical authorities.

## UTOPIAN EXEMPLARS

Within utopian communities a belief that commitment to a spiritual ideal, upright living, sobriety, and the proper form of sexuality (whose directives ranged from celibacy to free love) would forestall the intrusion of madness can be assumed. Though welcoming, let alone caring for, the mentally ill was not an agenda item, something certainly spilled over from the utopian communities into the homeopathic asylums. This was idealistic fervor, fastidious morality, and determination to be self-sufficient. Utopianism's heyday, when more than 100,000 disenchanted Americans sought to realize the ideal of a meaningful life, was 1820 to 1860. Yet the notion of a perfectly ordered community can be traced back to Plato's *Republic,* the book of Acts in the New Testament, and the works of Sir Thomas More in the sixteenth century. Even when not long lived, utopian communities served as invaluable incubators of social transformation. This perspective is powerfully expressed in *Utopia Method Vision: The Use Value of Social Dreaming* (Ralahine Utopian Studies).[1]

### Amana Society, New York

German emigrant Christian Metz, who was revered as a biblical prophet, led seven hundred people in establishing the self-sufficient Ebenezer Society community in 1843 in upstate New York as an instrument of the Community of True Inspiration, which had broken away from the Lutheran Church in Germany in 1714. The community relocated to Iowa in 1854 and established the Amana Society, where it expanded to seven villages over 25,000 acres. Families lived in individual houses but shared communal kitchens and dining halls. Amana celebrated the third centennial of the founding of the Community of True Inspiration in 2014.

### Brook Farm, Massachusetts

Transcendentalist writer and former Unitarian minister George Ripley founded Brook Farm Commune in 1841 to "prepare a society of liberal, intelligent, and cultivated persons whose relations with each other would permit a more wholesome and simple life than can be led amid the pressure of our competitive institutions." Few individuals actually lived on site early on, yet members strove to achieve self-sufficiency. In 1844, Brook Farm adopted a socialist constitution reflecting utopian socialist Charles Fourier's belief that people could live harmoniously under communal conditions and a republican-style government.* The commune suffered from lack of funds and fragmented after a new communal structure burned to the ground. It is remembered largely for the intellectual leaders and famous writers who resided there at various points in time, including Ralph Waldo Emerson and Nathaniel Hawthorne.

### New Harmony, Indiana

Wealthy industrialist Robert Owen believed that poverty would be eliminated if the unemployed could be collectivized within self-supporting villages. The commune he established in 1825 was based on the principles of the Enlightenment. His vision was a transformation of the social order, where social equality and individual enlightenment would be achieved by an emphasis on education and work. New Harmony's progressive ideas included an eight-hour workday, communal service, equal education for all, and equal rights and optional birth control for women.

### Oneida Community, New York

The Oneida Community was one of the most successful of its genre, founded in 1848 by a wealthy businessman who became a minister,

---

*Referring not to the Republican party but to elected representatives making laws serving a population's interests and advancing the common good.

John Humphrey Noyes. Noyes believed in perfectionism, the idea that religious conversion and willpower would release an individual from sin. He claimed that Christ had already returned to earth and that Jesus had commanded his followers to escape sin through faith in God, communal living, and polyamory. The Oneida Community numbered more than two hundred by 1851 and allowed that every man in the community was married to every woman and every woman to every man because "there is no more reason why sexual intercourse should be restrained by law, than why eating and drinking should be."

One of their members, a blacksmith named Sewell Newhouse, taught them how to hand-forge game traps, and the community developed and flourished commercially, selling not only traps but also silver flatware and other goods. In 1879, after local law officials attempted to arrest Noyes for adultery and his practice of polygamy, the community forsook universal marriage and converted to a joint stock company.

## Shakers

The Shakers, or Shaking Quakers, were pacifists who practiced communal living in the mid-1800s in eight states. At their peak the Shakers numbered more than six thousand members. Founder Ann Lee held that a genderless God was the female incarnation of the Trinity. So as to prepare her followers for heaven's perfection, she taught celibacy, and children were adopted rather than birthed. The Shakers communal farms manufactured and sold furniture and handicrafts, and commandeered the garden seed and medicinal herb businesses. Initially spontaneous dancing was a part of Shaker worship, which is how they got their name, but that was replaced by choreographed dancing before it eventually ceased. Shakers practiced social, sexual, economic, and spiritual equality for all members. Although appreciated for their enduring contribution to American crafts and architecture, the Shakers have dwindled to just two in a single village in Maine.

# AVATARS OF MORAL CARE, OR
# HUMANE TREATMENT

Prior to the eighteenth century, mental illness was more feared than understood, with scant advice or true help available. Often sufferers were locked away amid punishing conditions. Moral care emerged as a therapeutic approach that emphasized kindness with an intent to restore and build character. It derived from revulsion for existing barbaric treatment, spiritual and moral concern, and from the field of psychiatry's gradual concession that rather than be harshly judged the mentally ill's peculiar behaviors and narratives merited scrutiny.

## *Philippe Pinel*

Philippe Pinel served as physician of the infirmaries at Bicêtre, the men's public hospice near Paris, from 1793 to 1795. His famous 1794 *Memoir on Madness* conveys his "psychologic treatment" principles, a humane method for which he became known as the founder of French psychiatry. The revolutionary government constructed asylums where the mentally ill could be decently treated, maintaining that mental illness is often curable. Pinel maintained that to form a diagnosis the physician must carefully observe a patient's behavior, interview him, listen carefully, and document the interaction. Paramount to cure is understanding the natural history of the condition and its precipitating event. Only those patients who may be malicious or murderous require restraining. Pinel refined the work of Jean Baptiste Pussin, governor of the ward for the insane at Bicêtre public hospice who ordered removal of chains from the insane in 1797.[2]

## *William Tuke*

A reformist and philanthropist notable for his work in mental health, William Tuke was known for staunch Quaker principles he put into action. His work coincided with the emergence of similar work in France, most famously by Philippe Pinel in Paris and Samuel Hahnemann in Germany, as discussed in chapter 6.

Tuke, like so many others, was distressed by the torturous treatment King George III endured for his madness (initially attributed to porphyria, but it's now widely believed he was bipolar). His dismay was compounded by what he saw at York Lunatic Asylum in the spring of 1792, and he appealed to the Society of Friends (Quakers) to revolutionize treatment of the insane. By 1795, financial and social support from the community finally arrived when the Society of Friends eventually approved a plan suggesting raising funds through annuities. Tuke bought eleven acres of land and, in collaboration with a London architect, developed the new asylum called the York Retreat. The first of its kind in England, it pioneered more humane methods of treatment for the mentally ill.

While allowing physicians to observe and diagnose, Tuke forbade bleeding and other traditional "heroic" means of practice. Chains, manacles, and physical punishment were banned. Individualized treatment was based on benevolence, restoring self-esteem, and encouraging self-control among residents (who were not referred to as patients). The innovation of occupational therapy involving farm labor in peaceful surroundings was introduced. A social environment where residents were attached to a family-like unit built on kindness, moderation, order, and trust was developed. The facility had a spiritual dimension that involved prayer. Residents were permitted to choose their own clothing, encouraged to engage in handicrafts, to write, and to read books. Unlike other institutions at the time, York featured long, airy corridors that allowed patients to stroll, even if they were compelled to remain on the grounds. They were allowed to wander the retreat's courtyards and gardens, which were stocked with various small domestic animals.[3]

### Thomas Story Kirkbride

Another Quaker, Thomas Story Kirkbride, is memorable for his influential ideas about the design and construction of hospitals for the mentally ill. Kirkbride graduated from the University of Pennsylvania Medical School in 1832, and during his residency at a Quaker mental institution near Philadelphia he was able to witness moral treatment in action.

In 1841, Kirkbride became superintendent of the Pennsylvania

Hospital for the insane, which much later would become the Department for Mental and Nervous Diseases. At this newly founded hospital affiliated with the Pennsylvania Hospital, Kirkbride enjoyed sufficient administrative autonomy to design and install moral care treatment standards. Reduction in patient restraints was implemented, and a wide variety of recreational and educational activities were made available to patients.

Kirkbride's influential theories of hospital design and construction are put forth in his *On the Construction, Organization, and General Arrangements of Hospitals for the Insane* (1854). Those theories, which came to be known collectively as the Kirkbride Plan, called for a central building with wings projecting from it in a linear manner. The plan also called for no more than 250 residents (a principle later largely disregarded), with an ample, open campus surrounded by a large wall. Dozens of hospitals throughout the United States were built according to the Kirkbride Plan. Whether or not operational, many of the structures are still standing.

Remarkable among Kirkbride's innovations was his introduction of "magic lantern" shows into the institutional setting.

In the mid-1840s the field of photography was on the rise, providing Kirkbride with a technique to aid patients in overcoming their societal alienation. Kirkbride's belief was that the images would provide stability for patients by augmenting their visual perception, thereby correcting their understanding of the world outside of themselves. As the audience, patients would be part of "normal" social life, thus allowing for rational patterns of brain activity to take hold. With the new technology Kirkbride intended his magic lantern shows to serve as both therapy and entertainment for patients. The lantern itself was an early version of the slide projector, lit by candles and with slides inserted manually. Topics presented included astronomy, history, religion, and temperance. Travelogues were popular as well, simulating trips to Paris or London or around the corner to Philadelphia, and were accompanied by a lecturer offering commentary from a podium.[4]

In 1844, Kirkbride worked to co-create and later preside over the

Association of Medical Superintendents of American Institutions for the Insane (AMSAII).[5]

## The Example of Geel (formerly Gheel), Antwerp, Belgium

Since the thirteenth century, Geel has enjoyed renown as a nonjudgmental, non-stigmatizing haven for the mentally ill. The explanation comes via the hagiographic tale of Dymphna, a seventh-century Irish Christian princess who, oral tradition claimed, made a spiritual vow of chastity as a young teen. When her grief-addled, widowed father incestuously threatened that vow, Dymphna fled her homeland for Belgium, where she used her wealth to care for the sick, the poor, and particularly the mentally ill. Enraged to the point of madness, her father pursued and beheaded Dymphna in the year 600. In recognition of her martyrdom the princess was declared a saint, one with province over the mentally ill. The martyred princess is buried in a forest near the present site of Geel, where the Church of St. Dymphna was erected in her honor.

Dymphna's insurrection engendered her candidacy as a saint who could combat evil spirits, and pilgrims to Dymphna's tomb on behalf of those seen as possessed reported being rewarded with miraculous cures. As the Dymphna legend grew and Geel gained renown as a center for cures, village inhabitants and neighboring farmers started offering accommodation to mentally ill pilgrims who wished to remain and become productive citizens. Thus a nonmedical family foster care tradition arose. This development preceded the establishment of the first psychiatric hospital in the early fifteenth century in Valencia, Spain.

Upon admission the patient was observed for a brief period in the village infirmary before medical staff and Geel representatives decided on a plan of care. With group consensus the placement was made into a hand-selected family, with an 80 percent retention rate. The selection process that matched patients with family overseers required that the family have an upstanding reputation and an unblemished record with regard to legal issues. Certification entailed strong social standing and was also a long-established source of pride. The cost of family foster care was assumed by the patient's relatives or by the patient's community of origin.

The infirmary was utilized on the rare occasions when a patient became completely unmanageable. Upon restoration to a baseline state the patient was returned to the former boarding home. In the infrequent event that boarding-out was untenable, the patient was transferred to a sequestering mental institution.

The Catholic Church retained guardianship until 1852, when responsibility for its oversight was transferred to the state under medical direction.[6] It was during this phase of the project that Selden Talcott, while superintendent of Middletown Hospital, sojourned to Geel and returned to New York inspired by the program's implications for asylum care.

The heyday of the Geel guardianship program was just prior to World War II, when it represented the full range of mental health issues and included almost four thousand patients.

## A Model for the Future

While care for the mentally ill is still somewhat of an enigma, we know from these examples (and much of what follows in *Sane Asylums*) what works to the best benefit of the distressed and their families. Optimal care takes time and energy, in addition to the all-important concern of paying for it, and the public seems even less inclined today than two centuries ago to put their tax dollars in this direction.

*Sane Asylums* concludes with a vision of transformed mental health care for the future. It includes mental disorders shedding their stigma—not because we should be unashamed of disease states but in consideration of mental disorders being mostly a response to exigencies of the human condition. It foretells the necessity of a return to the foster care model of community care such as that seen in Geel; reliance on compassionate, holistically oriented caregivers; and abandonment of psychopharmacology-centered symptom suppression and of psychiatry's judgmental and contorted diagnostic lingo. If we are a compassionate people, we need to make this a priority.

# 3

## Homeopathy to the Fore

*Canst thou not minister to a mind diseased,*
*Pluck from the memory a rooted sorrow,*
*Raze out the written troubles of the brain,*
*And with some sweet oblivious antidote*
*Cleanse the stuff'd bosom of that perilous stuff*
*Which weighs upon the heart?*

WILLIAM SHAKESPEARE,
*MACBETH*, ACT V, SCENE 3

### SAMUEL HAHNEMANN

Samuel Christian Hahnemann (1755–1843) was a German physician educated at the universities of Leipzig, Vienna, and Erlangen. Disenchanted with the heroic medical practices of the day (bleeding, blistering, purging, and leeching), he proposed an alternative treatment regimen that combined nutritious food, clean air, and a concept known as the Law of Similars. The credo *Similia similibus curuntur* (let likes be cured by likes) restates what Hippocrates articulated in the fourth century BCE, that "medicines cure diseases similar to those they produce." Homeopathy expanded the principle's application. At the same time, the Law of Similars inadequately describes all that homeopathy does, since pathologies are cured that do not necessarily appear in the provings or in the toxicology profiles of the remedies.

---

## Homeopathic Drug Proving

The homeopathic drug proving process, also known as a Homeopathic Pathogenetic Trial, is a process that puts drugs on trial by having healthy human volunteers ingest a non-dilute amount and, over a period of weeks or months, having been kept ignorant of the substance's identity, noting its pathogenic effect. This is the first step to including a drug composed of a highly diluted and succussed (vigorously shaken, thereby potentized) form of the original substance in the homeopathic materia medica (materials of medicine), a reference guide that lists curative indications and therapeutic actions of homeopathic medicines.

---

In dilute form, remedies made from herbs simply enhance the action of the herb. In many instances homeopathic and allopathic medicine actions overlap (see the discussion of David Dyce Brown's book, *The Permeation of Present Day Medicine by Homoeopathy,* in chapter 4). Modern and better explanations of homeopathy's systemic effect are now at hand. In the appendix section you'll find a discussion of psychiatrist Iris Bell's research indicating that homeopathy promotes the body's ability to achieve homeostasis.

Hahnemann's belief that a medicinal agent discloses its essence via its "proving" within a healthy individual remains weighty. Symptoms released in the proving reflect the vital powers and uniqueness of the organism. An ill person presenting with a certain set of symptoms as a result of disease can have that disease cured by administration of the *similar* developed by the proving. The similar is a much diluted and potentized (via succussion, or vigorous shaking) solution of the substance that in a gross amount inculcates in a healthy person those very same symptoms. In the homeopathic view, symptoms represent the body's natural defense process at work fighting the disease, not the disease itself.

Hahnemann's 1792 intervention was both a brilliant success and a paradigm example of nonjudgmental, scrupulous observation,

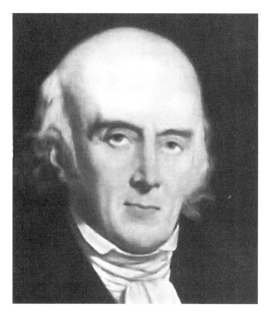

Samuel Hahnemann

diagnosis, and treatment. He was a great pioneer in replacing brutality with psychologically oriented moral care in the treatment of the mentally ill.

Hahnemann's major work conveying these subtle notions was his seminal work, the *Organon,* the first edition of which appeared in 1810 under a German title that translates to "Organon of rational medicine." It was revised repeatedly and published with slight name changes in six different editions (five during his lifetime).

During his long career Hahnemann relocated several times in Europe, and by the late 1830s he was living in Paris and had become famous. Long lines of carriages, many carrying the aristocracy of the continent, regularly lined up outside Hahnemann's sumptuous residence, often waiting as long as three hours for an appointment. Assisting him in his extensive case taking (see the accounts on the following pages) was his wife Melanie; under the master's supervision she prescribed for the dozens of impoverished patients who throughout the day gathered outside the gates. Poverty-stricken patients were not charged, and Hahnemann billed paying patients only if a cure was achieved.

## THE CURE OF F. A. KLOCKENBRING

Toward the end of 1791 or the beginning of 1792, when Samuel Hahnemann was residing in Gotha, Germany, his friend R. Z. Becker, editor and proprietor of a newspaper called the *Reichanzeiger*, at Hahnemann's suggestion wrote an article proposing the creation of an asylum utilizing gentle methods to treat the upper-class insane. The article caught the attention of the wife of Friedrich A. Klockenbring, the dissolute Hanoverian minister of police and secretary to the chancellery. Herr Klockenbring was said to have lost his mind due to overwork and his "fast life." This resulted in his being targeted in a satiric media attack portraying him as intimate with drunken brothel keepers and possessed of "the most dangerous venereal disease, and moral vices ranging from drunkenness to fraud." A man of stature for whom public standing and self-respect were paramount, the hugely affronted Klockenbring had deteriorated (his symptoms were those of the tertiary stages of syphilis) to where he was adjudged violently insane.

In June 1792 he was brought to Georgenthal in so aggressive a state as to warrant escort and restraint by two burly men. His face, covered with large spots, was described as filthy and imbecilic in expression. He was afflicted with strange hallucinations and babbled in Greek and Hebrew. In his excitable mania Klockenbring destroyed his clothing and bedding and smashed his piano into pieces. Day and night the ravings continued.

Duke Ernst of Saxe-Gotha gave over to Hahnemann a wing of his hunting castle nearby, mandating that the doctor establish a mental asylum there. Situated in a beautiful area at the foot of the Thuringian Forest not far from the capital city of Gotha, the institution opened in August 1792. Hahnemann's lengthy account illustrates his objectivity, compassion, and keenness of observation.

*Hither the privy secretary of the chancer, Herr Klockenbring, of Hanover, who lately died from the effects of a surgical operation in the 53d year of his age, was brought and placed under my care.*

*He was a man who in his days of health attracted the admiration of a large portion of Germany by his practical talents for business and his profound sagacity, as also by his knowledge of ancient and modern lore, and his acquirements in various branches of science. His almost superhuman labours in the department of state police, for which he had a great talent, his constant sedentary life, the continued strain upon his mind, together with a too nutritious diet [and] his copious indulgence in strong wines contributed to bring on this state. . . . His mind, that was almost too sensitive to honour and fair fame, sank deep into the dust beneath this hail-storm of abusive accusations. . . .*

*At first he ran about and bellowed, mostly at night. He exhibited a great inclination to dress himself up, so as to give himself an amazingly majestic or half heroic, half Merry-Andrew-like [clownish] appearance. . . . Smiles and grinding of the teeth, inconsiderateness and insolence, cowardice and defiance, childish folly and unlimited pride, desires without wants. His bloated body, which in his days of health was somewhat unwieldy, now exhibited a wondrous agility, quickness and flexibility in all its movements.*

*Incessantly, day and night, he kept on raving, and was never composed for a quarter of an hour at a time. When he sank down exhausted on his bed, he rose to his feet again in a few minutes [with] threatening gestures, [suggesting] capital sentences on criminals, . . . and spouted, as [the warriors] Agamemnon and Hector, entire passages from the* Iliad *then he would whistle a popular song, roll about on the grass. For the first fortnight I only observed him without treating him medicinally.*

*Spoke in the exact words of the Hebrew text; but he finished nothing that he began, for some new idea constantly led him into a different region; he would burst forth in an agony of weeping and sobbing, often throwing himself at the feet of the amazed attendant, write magical characters on the sand at his feet, make the sign of the cross, then he would burst out into immoderate fits of laughter, his piano to pieces and setting it together again in an absurd manner. The most wonderful thing was the correctness with which he delivered all the passages from writings in all languages that occurred to his memory, especially all that he had learnt in his youth.[1]*

Period of Convalescence

*As he began to improve, this faculty of divination [in addition to using unfamiliar languages and spouting precise literary passages, he wrote a detailed prescription despite his lack of medical education] became always more and more vague and uncertain, until at last, when his reason was completely restored, he knew neither more nor less about the matter than other people. . . . I begged him, in a friendly manner, to explain this enigma to me . . . "I shudder and a cold chill comes all over me," he replied, "when I think about it; I must beg of you not to remind me of this subject."*

*His friendship, which I enjoyed for two years after his complete restoration, has richly repaid me for these and thousands of other sad moments I passed on his account.*

*Before he quitted my establishment he shewed to the public, by his translation of a statistical work of [agriculturist] Arthur Young, his regenerated intelligence in a very advantageous manner, and after he quitted me the government of his native land bestowed on him, in place of his former too toilsome office, the direction of the lottery, which he continued to hold till his death.*

*Peace be with his ashes!*

## *Hahnemann's Remedy Choice*

According to Jütte, this report issues from a mixture of extracts from *The Lesser Writings of Samuel Hahnemann* and Richard Haehl's biography, *Samuel Hahnemann: His Life & Work,* both in English translation that corresponds with a 1796 account that appeared in the journal *Deutsche Monatsschrift.*

*At last Hahnemann reached his decision as to which of his remedies would help Klockenbring. He gave a single dose of Antimonium tartaricum. Within six months Klockenbring had recovered sufficiently to enter the world. Again, Hahnemann didn't have any "remedies" at the time—he didn't begin doing provings and recording symptoms until several years hence. Hahnemann was treating his patient with no medicine, a good dose of compassion, and changes in hygiene and diet. At one point the patient began to eat to the point of gluttony and Hahnemann prescribed "25 grains" [approximately 1.6 grams] of tartar emetic (Ant. tart.) to help the patient vomit. That was his only drug prescription.*[2]

From my own perspective as a longtime practitioner of homeopathy: In regard to gluttony, Antimonium crudum would be the more appropriate choice. One marvels at the choice of Antimonium tartaricum. In fact, numerous other remedies are at hand in which the symptom of overeating is prominent. What Hahnemann pinpointed in his scrupulous method, early on in the development of homeopathy, was a subtle feature of Klockenbring—namely, an extreme touchiness evident in Klockenbring's susceptibility to an affront. Ant. tart. in my practice comes up most usually for children exhibiting this touchiness, a tendency to take things personally. Klockenbring's cure in large part comes down to Hahnemann's subtle perception that because his patient was touchy, Antimonium tartaricum was indicated. While it would be an oversimplification to say that it cured the entire case, Hahnemann's prescription was a permission slip offering Klockenbring's vital force the opportunity to release itself from the underlying delusion that an affront is the end of the world.

Hahnemann holds in common with doctors of traditional Chinese medicine that the presence of emotional and mental disturbance does not require a separate and distinct category of pathology. He would not have been impressed by the emergence of psychiatry or the modern era's psychopharmacology.

Hahnemann's thoughts concerning mental imbalance are scattered around all six editions of the *Organon*. Those wishing to encounter his words directly can explore these texts, but attend especially to aphorisms 117 and 210–30 (summaries are given in chapter 6 and the full aphorisms in the appendices).

All homeopathic materia medica texts (references describing the full range of action for substances utilized for medical purposes) feature a prominent mind section in which rubrics listing delusions receive such close attention that the pages become dog-eared from use. Indeed, rare would be the patient visiting a homeopath for whom "delusions of the mind" does not come into play. So if we are all deluded does this mean we are all mentally ill? Or does it indicate that being human entails possessing a behavioral susceptibility, entrenched notion, or everyday fear that, when extenuated, simply gets out of hand? In the case of

A. F. Klockenbring, madness is deconstructed as centered on a touchiness that has mushroomed into terror and confusion.

## EARLY PURVEYORS OF
## HOMEOPATHY TO AMERICA

Though they likely did not know of one another, two students of Hahnemann planted the seeds of homeopathy in America in divergent locations at essentially the same time: German physician William Wesselhoeft, who arrived at the borough of Bath, Pennsylvania, in 1824, and Danish physician Hans Burch Gram, who taught homeopathy to conventional medicine colleagues in New York in 1825.

### William Wesselhoeft

In 1824, Dr. William Wesselhoeft, an avid herbalist, arrived from Germany and soon became the recipient of homeopathic books and medicines from a Hahnemann disciple, Dr. John Ernst Stapf.[3]

One of his students, Rev. Johannes Helffrich, considered the father of the German Reformed Church in America, was caught up in Wesselhoeft's passion for homeopathic medicine and created a botanical garden, hothouse, and laboratory at his parsonage. He, Wesselhoeft, and Swiss physician Henry Detwiller formed a homeopathic study group.

The practitioners gained renown, and an enlargement of the facilities became necessary. In 1828, Rev. Helffrich built the house that still stands today in the Borough of Bath, where the first homeopathic hospital in the United States was established. At a school operated in conjunction with the hospital, Rev. Helffrich was among the first to receive a degree.

Dr. Wesselhoeft later went to Philadelphia, where he founded the Hahnemann Hospital and Medical School.

Rev. Helffrich subsequently became one of the founders of the North American Academy of the Homeopathic Healing Art, also known as the Allentown Academy. As they constitute a precious record of homeopathy's inception and growth in America, Helffrich's medical effects are retained by the Smithsonian Institute in Washington.

Dissolved in 1841, the Allentown Academy was replaced by

the Homeopathic Medical College of Pennsylvania in 1848, with Dr. Constantine Hering as one of its founders.[4]

### *Hans Burch Gram*

In 1823, Danish physician Hans Burch Gram took up studies with Hans Christian Lund, the earliest and most prominent Danish homeopath, who may have been a student of Hahnemann. Like the great physician and teacher James Tyler Kent, he was a follower of the mystical philosopher Emanuel Swedenborg. Swedenborg's influence on American Transcendentalists spilled over into medicine. Through his message "As above (the realm of heaven), so below (the realm of earth)," Swedenborg supported high-dilution (potency) remedies as a means of treating illness rooted in spiritual malaise. Gram would go on to become known as a godfather of American homeopathy.

In 1825, Dr. Gram returned to America, where he was swindled and suffered a financial loss that required his resumption of medical practice. Optimistic that the new homeopathic method could gain traction, he published his translation of Hahnemann's "Spirit of the Homeopathic Doctrine" essay in 1825.

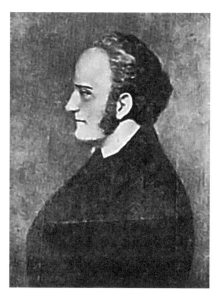

Hans Burch Gram

Gram gained the acquaintance of a fellow Mason and medical colleague, Robert B. Folger, who in 1826 read Gram's pamphlet. After initially being skeptical of homeopathy, Folger allowed Gram to treat several of his patients, these being among the first homeopathic patients in America. Impressed with the patients' recoveries, Folger took up the study of German to better read Hahnemann's work, and became Gram's student and assistant.[5]

Folger introduced Gram to Ferdinand Wilsey, who became one of his early patients when treatment of his "inveterate dyspepsia" by his allopathic doctor, John Gray, floundered.[6] Where Gray had failed, Gram succeeded. Still not fully convinced that Gram's methods had been effective, Gray created a trial in which Gram would treat additional difficult cases.

In Dr. Gray's own words:

*Gram's inimitable modesty in debate, and his earnest zeal for the good and the true in all ways and directions, and his vast culture in science and art, in history and philosophy, greatly surpassing in these respects any of the academic or medical professors I had known, very much shortened my dialectic opposition to the new system.*

*I selected three cases for the trial: the first, haemoptysis [coughing of blood] in a scrofulous [tuberculosis or similar bacteria of the lymph nodes, particularly of the neck] girl, complicated with amenorrhoea; the second, mania puerperalis [post-partum depression] of three months' standing; and the last, anasarca [extreme generalized edema] and ascites [abdominal swelling] in an habitual drunkard.*

*Following Gram's instructions, I furnished the proper registry of the symptoms in each case. He patiently and faithfully waded through the six volumes of Hahnemann's Materia Medica (luckily we had no manuals then), and prescribed a single remedy in each case.*

*The first and third cases were promptly cured by a single dose of the remedy prescribed, and the conditions as to diet and moral impressions were so arranged by me (Gram did not see either of the patients) that, greatly to my surprise and joy, very little room was left for a doubt as to the efficacy of the specifics applied.*

*The case of mania was perhaps the stronger testimony of the two. The patient was placed under the rule of diet for fourteen days previous to the administration of the remedy chosen by Gram.*

*Not the slightest mitigation of the maniacal sufferings occurred at that time. At the time of the giving of the remedy, which was a single drop of very dilute tincture of Nux vomica in a drink of sweetened water, the patient was more furious than usual, tearing her clothing off and angrily resisting all attempts to soothe her. She fully recovered her reason within half an hour after taking the Nux vomica, and never lost it afterwards.[7]*

As our topic is mental illness, a word about Nux vomica in relation to mania is in order. This is a remedy for type A personalities, furious multitaskers who claim they crave a moment of peace, but due to their need for control, they experience life as a constant battle. One of the greatest contributors to homeopathic literature was Baron Clemens Maria Franz von Boenninghausen, who in 1803 published a renowned cure for an otherwise—and to this day untreatable—condition: cholera. According to von Boenninghausen's character designation of the remedy:

Great anxiety and restlessness in evening. Immoderately anxious scrupulosity. Zealous, fiery temperament. Quarrelsome. Malicious, spiteful disposition. Inclination to reproach others. Surly, refractory mood. Easily startled. Violent and excitable. Suicidal thoughts; when looking at a knife he is inclined to stab himself, when at water, to drown himself, yet he fears death. Insanity of drunkards. Oversensitive to external impressions. Time passes too slowly. Moroseness.[8]

Note: all of these symptoms are produced from a proving of the original Nux vomica substance—poison nut, or strychnine tree.

Seeing these patients flourishing under Gram's care converted Gray, who then transitioned into homeopathy and a successful New York practice. He became an effective homeopathic emissary within New York's neighboring states, as well as editor of the *American Journal of*

*Homeopathy* and the *Homœopathic Examiner,* the latter a journal of the Hahnemann Medical College of Philadelphia.

Hans Gram's position as president of the New York Medical and Philosophical Society gained him respect and influence over a number of physicians. Their conversion to homeopathic practice and subsequent success in treating victims of the cholera epidemic of 1832 propelled New York City into a homeopathic mecca. By and by these physicians would spread the doctrine of Hahnemann throughout not only New York state but also Massachusetts, Connecticut, and New Jersey. Gram's mentorship of the pioneering homeopathic cadre continued until his death in 1840.

## HOMEOPATHIC ASSOCIATIONS AND MEDICAL SCHOOLS

In 1844 the American Institute of Homeopathy (AIH) was founded by homeopathic physicians from New York, Philadelphia, and Boston. It was the first national medical organization in the United States, established to promote standardization of the practice and teaching of homeopathy.

### Conventional Medicine Strikes Back

The American Institute of Homeopathy preceded any formal association of allopaths (conventional physicians). Partly in response to this alliance, in 1847 allopathic physicians founded the American Medical Association (AMA) (see the introduction concerning the AMA's pecuniary motivation). In 1855 the AMA codified its fear of homeopathy by installing its infamous non-consultation clause, according to which members were enjoined from consulting (or even socializing) with homeopathic physicians. The AMA chose to drop the non-consultation clause in 1901, not because the association was no longer opposed to homeopathy, but because it had discovered more effective methods of defeating it.

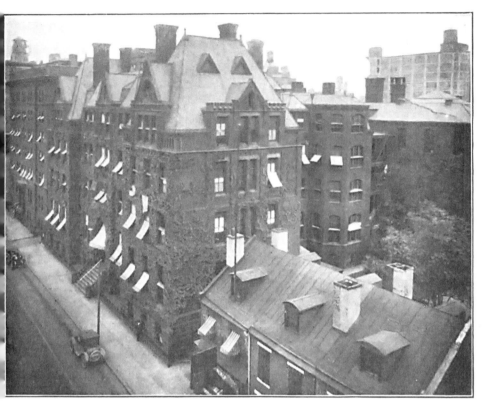

**Hahnemann Hospital and Medical College, Philadelphia**
Courtesy of the American Institute of Homeopathy, from *Hospitals and Sanatoriums of the Homoeopathic School of Medicine* (1916)

By 1848 twelve homeopathic medical colleges existed in the United States, among them Boston's New England Female Medical College. Founded by Dr. Israel Tilsdale Talbot, the school was revolutionary for empowering women in a male-dominated field. It became the first institution in the United States to train women in medicine and graduated the first black female physician, Rebecca Lee Crumpler. In 1873 it merged with Boston University, becoming the first accredited coeducational medical school in the United States, and continued to teach homeopathic medicine well into the twentieth century.

In 1867, Constantine Hering withdrew from the Homeopathic Medical College of Pennsylvania that he had cofounded, and founded the Hahnemann Medical College of Philadelphia, which later merged with the Homeopathic Medical College of Pennsylvania. That in turn eventually merged with another visionary school, the Woman's Medical College, which had originally started as the Female Medical College of Pennsylvania in 1850.

In Pennsylvania, over time the Hahnemann Medical College and the Woman's Medical College of Pennsylvania would evolve into Drexel University College of Medicine, College of Nursing and Health Professions, and Dornsife School of Public Health.

# 4

---------

# The Madness of
# Mary Todd Lincoln

*If I must die,*
*I will encounter darkness as a bride,*
*And hug it in mine arms.*

WILLIAM SHAKESPEARE,
*MEASURE FOR MEASURE*, ACT III, SCENE 1

Two schools of thought contend over the madness and recovery from madness of President Abraham Lincoln's widow, Mary. The first suggests that she was railroaded into a court hearing on her state of mind and subsequent finding of insanity by the efforts of her greedy son and heir, Robert. According to this narrative Mary Lincoln was actually not in need of treatment, and her liberation from the injustice of indefinite confinement in a mental asylum can be credited to her wily legal advisers, James and Myra Bradwell. According to the second school of thought, Mary Lincoln was genuinely insane and a huge concern to her loving son Robert. In this narrative all she needed to recover her wits was a sojourn out of the public eye, a dose of peace and quiet.

These many years later, a third narrative is introduced.

## A WOMAN CHARMING, OUTGOING, AND AMBITIOUS

Mary was an engaging if erratic personality as well as a nervous, impulsive woman prone to extravagant spending and grandiosity. Yet, after her second son, Edward, died in 1850 at the tender age of three, Mary began to exhibit depressive symptoms that deepened when, soon after, she was thrown from a moving vehicle and concussed. Her rehabilitation required several weeks.

In the wake of her widowhood she had to endure a humiliating and highly public betrayal. William H. Herndon, Lincoln's law partner and biographer, initiated a popular lecture series that suggested Lincoln had never recovered from the untimely death of his first love, Anne Rutledge, who had been betrothed to another man, and thus knew no joy during his twenty-three years of marriage to Mary. This false

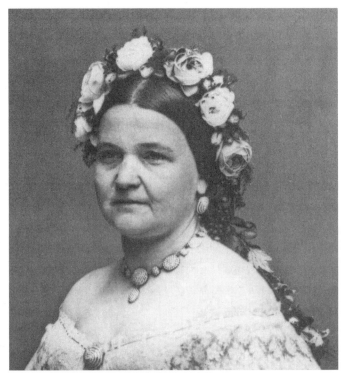

Mary Todd Lincoln

Victorian-era trope depicting Mary as a "female wild cat of the age" infected historians' views of her for years to come.

In quest of relief from her psychic pain Mary turned to spiritualism as a means of communicating with her two deceased children—Eddie, who died of tuberculosis, and Willie, who succumbed to cholera or possibly typhoid fever. Surprisingly, although her husband was a lawyer he left no will to be executed upon his death. The several years it took for the family finances to be sorted and monies distributed were yet another stress on Mary, contributing to financial strain and fears of impoverishment, homelessness, fire, and theft. A breaking point for her son Robert was when Mary, gripped by her tormenting delusions and preparing to vacate the White House, sought to sell some of the ball gowns she could no longer wear as a widow, thus rendering her a public laughingstock and mortifying her son.

## HOMEOPATHY AND THE LINCOLN FAMILY

Abraham Lincoln and his family were devotees of homeopathy. At the outset of his legal career in 1854, Lincoln lobbied and prepared to develop a special legislative charter for a homeopathic medical school in Chicago. According to researchers Allen D. Spiegel and Florence Kavaler:

> Animosity between allopathic or orthodox medical practitioners and irregular healers made this no picnic. The economic success of homeopathic practitioners infuriated conventional physicians, a situation their nascent American Medical Association was formed to combat. In addition, the poor reputation of medical education in the United States generally rendered the project non-compelling. But Lincoln's allies included Chicago's mayor, two congressmen, an Illinois state representative, a Chicago city councilman, the co-founder of Northwestern University, the founder of Chicago Union Railroad, and several medical doctors themselves homeopaths. Lincoln and his team secured the charter, thereby midwifing into

existence the Hahnemann Homeopathic Medical College, whose first class was admitted in 1860, whereafter the school remained in existence for almost sixty-five years.[1]

President Lincoln associated himself with homeopathic advocates. These included the postmaster general, the secretary of the treasury, and his most trusted adviser, Secretary of State William Seward. Salmon P. Chase, Lincoln's Secretary of the Treasury, may have had his life saved by homeopathy after being treated for cholera in the summer of 1849, when a cholera epidemic was rampant. Montgomery Blair, Lincoln's postmaster general, was the head of the National Homeopathic Hospital in Washington, D.C.

If you visit the Pearson Museum at Southern Illinois University you will see an exhibit of a nineteenth-century doctor's office and drug store that includes a homeopathic medicine kit from the Diller Drug Store of Springfield, Illinois, where Abraham Lincoln was a frequent customer. The Lincoln Financial Foundation Collection has, courtesy of the Indiana State Museum, a pen and ink sketch by artist and historian Lloyd Ostendorf depicting Abraham Lincoln with druggist Roland Weaver Diller at the Corneau-Diller Drug Store. Lincoln's arm rests on the counter behind which stands pharmacist Diller in a white coat preparing to weigh something on the scale.

Mrs. Lincoln was a long-standing patient of Dr. Willis Danforth, a homeopathic surgeon who prescribed for her migraine headaches and insomnia. After homeopathy successfully cured her sciatica, a condition that had resisted all manner of allopathic remedies for more than six weeks, Danforth became converted to its practice, openly espousing allegiance to homeopathy in 1860. In October 1869, Danforth was elected professor of surgery in the Hahnemann Medical College, locating there the following spring. He was elected president of the Chicago Academy of Medicine, became associate editor of the *United States Medical and Surgical Journal,* and was surgeon in chief to Scammon Hospital, Chicago. He provided testimony at Mary Lincoln's first hearing to the effect that she was insane.[2]

In 1999 the *Chicago Tribune* reported that a trove of letters written by Mrs. Lincoln to Dr. Danforth in the 1870s while she was living in Chicago were sold by Danforth's descendants to the Henry Horner Lincoln Collection. Included was a letter to Danforth beseeching him to provide her relief from headaches, requesting that he send "about four more powders—I had a miserable night last night and took the five you left." Curator Kim Bauer of the Illinois Historical Library states, "the exact medication is unknown."[3]

Though low-potency homeopathic drugs such as Danforth prescribed may be repeated, they do not addict. Under no circumstance would Dr. Danforth, a homeopathic physician and recognized homeopathic authority, have subjected his patient to allopathic, dependency-fostering patent medicines. That it was homeopathics Mary Lincoln sought from her physician is more than likely.

On the infamous night when Lincoln was assassinated, a Booth co-conspirator, Lewis Powell, entered the home of Secretary of State William Seward with the idea of assassinating high government officials to throw the federal government into chaos. He had gained entry by claiming to have a delivery of medicines from Seward's homeopathic doctor, Tullio S. Verdi, M.D. Conjunct with Lincoln's murder, Seward too was a victim at the theater, stabbed in the anti-Union plot.[4]

## MENTAL HEALTH AND
## TRIAL OF MARY TODD LINCOLN

Mary Lincoln had a tragic history whose culmination in insanity has been attributed to numerous causes. These include diabetes, pernicious anemia, grief, and a brain tumor found upon autopsy. She was also dependent on a variety of prescription medicines, including a sedative for her persistent insomnia, chloral hydrate, which is associated with severe withdrawal syndrome and may induce liver damage.

From a homeopathic standpoint, determinants were psychological blows relating to unbearable grief over the premature deaths of two of her four sons; the trauma of her unpopularity due to having grown up in the Confederate South; the assassination of her husband, Abraham Lincoln; losing three half brothers and a brother-in-law in the Civil

War; and the actual or perceived enmity of her surviving son, Robert, who ultimately had his mother institutionalized.

Abraham Lincoln's confession to his biographer, friend, and law partner of eighteen years, William Herndon, that he was infected with syphilis in 1835 or 1836 is also significant. Herndon, believing both Mary Todd and Abraham Lincoln had syphilis, suspected it in the premature death of three Lincoln children;[5] two of them are believed to have died of tuberculosis, which is hastened by syphilis. Mary Lincoln's blindness in later life also suggests syphilitic pathology. For more information about syphilis as an inheritable liability, see *syphilitic diathesis* (particular type of suffering) in appendix 1, "Compendium of Madness Perspectives."

At her trial it was said that

> Mary claimed to hear voices through the walls; servants were forced to stand guard over their fearful mistress while she slept. Her alternating habits of wasteful spending and frugal saving were exposed before the court. Speculation concerning whether Mrs. Lincoln should or could have been diagnosed with syphilis, psychosis, pernicious anemia, bipolar depression, or schizophrenia continues unabated.
>
> One of Mary's doctors, Willis Danforth, was the star witness. He reported that Mary had told him that an evil Indian spirit was pulling wires out of her left eye, that she was distracted by premonitions of her own death, and that she was prone to vomiting up her meals to foil imaginary poisoners. The manager of the Chicago hotel she lived in explained how Mary had shown up in the elevator half-naked, and sent all her belongings to Milwaukee one day believing the city was being consumed by a raging fire.[6]

## IN THE CARE OF RICHARD J. PATTERSON

Upon a finding of insanity by a court, a request by the Lincoln family resulted in the unfortunate fifty-six-year-old paranoid and suicidal woman being remanded to institutional care.[7] Consulted on Robert Lincoln's behalf together with a Lincoln family friend and other familiar physicians, Danforth endorsed the choice of Richard J. Patterson, a physician reputedly expert in the progressive treatment of mental illness.

On what expertise did Dr. Patterson's reputation rest? Available information indicates that his practice involved compassionate (moral) care and a family patronage model such as was practiced in Geel, Belgium, where respect and tolerance for the insane individual was valued. Justifying the esteem in which Patterson was held, he likely had better cards to play.

What Patterson accomplished in the course of treating Mrs. Lincoln for a mere three months is eye opening. While at Bellevue the supposedly incurable Mary succeeded in living a normal life. "She visited with the superintendent's wife, took rides in her carriage, talked to the Pattersons' retarded daughter Blanche, and sat on the front stairs and wrote letters."[8]

The regain of her wherewithal together with the aid of lawyers enabled Mary to engineer her release from indefinite confinement. Once she'd gained her freedom, one of Mrs. Lincoln's attorneys told a Chicago newspaper reporter: "Mary Lincoln is no more insane than I am." Mary left Bellevue Place on September 11, 1875, when she was released into the custody of her sister, Elizabeth Edwards. On June 15, 1876, Mary Todd Lincoln was officially declared sane in a Chicago court.[9]

The scrolls documenting Dr. Patterson's methods regarding Mary Lincoln or other Bellevue patients may be missing, but circumstantial evidence indicates that his sanatorium at Bellevue Place in Batavia, Illinois, operating contemporaneously with the famed Middletown Hospital, was a kindred sane asylum. Bellevue boasted a greenhouse, orchards, vegetable garden, laundry facility, stables, and smoke- and icehouses, and Patterson was rumored to use gentle medicines popular at the time.[10] Other than homeopathics, what could those have been?

Patterson graduated from Berkshire Medical College in 1842 and was an administratively adept, upwardly mobile, and ultimately prosperous physician. After a stint as assistant physician in the State

Lunatic Hospital of Ohio he became medical superintendent of the Central Indiana Hospital for the Insane (a Kirkbride Moral Treatment center); he later was the first to supervise the Iowa State Insane Asylum. Simultaneous with this he held an appointment as superintendent of the Ohio Asylum for the Education of Idiotic and Imbecile Youth.[11] Patterson and his wife had a mentally disabled daughter, Blanche, and this may have enlarged his capacity for compassionate rendering to compromised individuals.

Patterson also served as professor of medical jurisprudence in Chicago Medical School. The clause in the Illinois law for the commitment of the insane, providing for the appointment of a medical commission by a judge of the court in lieu of a jury trial, was entirely his doing.

Antebellum physicians such as Patterson, but also Selden Talcott, agreed that insanity was a disease of the brain. It was sometimes true but often surmised that examination of brain tissue would reveal organic or functional abnormalities; that brain hemorrhage, tissue lesions, or indirect diseases such as suppression of the menses or pulmonary disease over time could damage the central nervous system and the brain.

It was conceded that the cause of cerebral disease could also be moral, meaning issuing from physical, cultural, economic, or spiritual stresses. Thus, in an era before scientific medicine was to wreak havoc on patients' well-being, moral care and homeopathic physicians could reasonably attribute insanity to a host of social problems. These could include domestic abuse, "Mexican War excitement," Millerism (a religious sect founded on the belief that God's wrath would descend upon the earth before the millennium), and frustration with the unattainable dream of greater rights for the common man promulgated by Jacksonian democracy. While postulating neurological dysfunction, such doctors respected the human mind along with the existential battles it waged and did not always win. Psychiatry's mad quest to reengineer the brain was not yet at hand.

## OVERLAPPING OF CONVENTIONAL
## AND HOMEOPATHIC MEDICINE
## IN THE MID- TO LATE-NINETEENTH CENTURY

Though his pedigree was allopathic, the argument that Richard Patterson used homeopathy to quickly render Mary Todd Lincoln mentally stable is indicated by:

- the congruence of the Batavia Institute and Middletown State Homeopathic Hospital for the insane with regard to Thomas Kirkbride moral treatment orientation, abundant greenery, and loveliness of surroundings;
- Mary Lincoln's referral to Dr. Patterson's care by at least one well-known homeopath;
- homeopathy was at its zenith in 1875, the year Mary Lincoln arrived at Bellevue, and the same fervor for homeopathy had propelled the funding and development of Middletown Hospital, which opened its doors in 1874;
- Patterson's shrewdness in maintaining conventional-medicine credibility, and his ability to operate in rarified administrative heights while reserving for himself utilization of popular medicines (read homeopathics), a protective ruse enabling his reputation as master of madness (unaccountable by purely moral treatment means) to be fostered; and
- the remarkable outcome of Mary Lincoln's gain of wherewithal occurring within four months of her unrecorded care from Dr. Patterson.

To these we append another compelling argument. In a non-regulatory era before professional boundaries were mapped, respected, or enforced, the practice of conventional medicine and homeopathy overlapped. This was not surprising since all physicians, not just homeopaths, retained the prerogative to control the level of dilution of medicines they would themselves compound.

A complex case might challenge a physician with contradictory features, such as when a chronically weak patient generally in need of support had a crisis that produced acute symptoms needing immediately to be subdued. A physician in this situation, especially one trying to adjust the concentration level of his medicine, could prescribe an "incorrect" medicine only to stumble upon a homeopathic effect. This he would either brush off as a meaningless anomaly (so much for scientific curiosity) or congratulate himself for having made an apparently brilliant discovery. Doctrine constrained him from admitting a universal principle, the Law of Similars (an example of which we'll see shortly), in action.

Since both they and their patients benefited, many physicians did not openly deny homeopathy's power. Yet the fruit could not be resisted. Were Richard Patterson's poaching from the neighboring orchard openly done, he would have been ostracized from the medical profession. He kept no records of his methods of treatment. Territorial rivalry was a high-stakes game.

Weary of hypocrisy, a homeopathic British physician, Dr. David Dyce Brown, finally called time-out. Come on guys, he in effect said, Who are you kidding?[12]

Dr. Brown's 1904 book (begun in 1867) and commissioned by the British Homeopathic Association is informatively titled *The Permeation of Present-Day Medicine by Homeopathy*. In it the author painstakingly details a hypocrisy: while not deigning to recognize Samuel Hahnemann, the founder of homeopathy, his immense body of work, or homeopathy itself, authoritative texts penned by conventional medical authors of the time vaingloriously displayed the action of seventy-two medicines common to both systems precisely as the same drugs are portrayed in homeopathic literature. The authorities' doubletalk bespoke a preferred reality in which the hard-won knowledge homeopaths possess is there for the taking, but the homeopathic practitioners themselves have been wished into nonexistence. Brown pointed out that though imitation may be the sincerest form of flattery, it is also unscrupulous. The animosity of the society of conventional medicine and the thievery of its authorities is not to be explained away.

Our friends of the old school [conventional medicine], while running down our principles of treatment as unscientific, call us the "grave of medicine," term us "absurd" while refusing to meet us in consultation and preventing us becoming members of the various medical societies, or holding any public appointments in connection with hospitals or otherwise; while calling themselves "regular" practitioners, and us, consequently, irregular ones—in other words, professionally tabooing us; . . . . yet they "show clearly how our principles and practice are adopted by them, though without any acknowledgment or any hint of the source from which the "new" treatment is obtained.[13]

Brown goes on to point out that in a typical excerpt like this we find the homeopathic wheel reinvented.

Elsewhere I have tried to show that a drug may fulfill various purposes, according to the doses in which it is given, and according to the times in which it is administered. A small quantity may do one sort of good, and a larger quantity another sort of good; and these two results may be not only quite different, but even of a contrary kind. Thus *ipecacuanha* [Ipecac] is a typical emetic when administered in the quantity of (say) 4 fluid drachms [three-fourths teaspoon] of the wine; but 1- or 2-drop doses of the same preparation given every hour have a growing reputation for the power of arresting sickness.[14]

What Brown is pointing out is that physicians in actual practice noticed that ipecacuana in a gross amount provoked vomiting but when diluted (homeopathic Ipecac) ameliorated the nausea. However they could not bring themselves to credit homeopathic principles for this relationship between a highly dilute (and thereby, homeopathic) substance and its beneficial action.

Along with thousands of others, in 1871, Mary Lincoln fell victim to the popularity of chloral hydrate. A highly addictive drug, also known as chloral, it was used to treat insomnia. Chloral hydrate acts as a depressant on the central nervous system, producing a sedative effect. Had Dr. Patterson encountered the following passages found in the April 8, 1871, issue of *The Lancet* (a renowned conventional medicine journal), he almost certainly would have recognized the drug's full-dose danger and might have considered treating Mary Lincoln with a homeopathic dose of the same drug.

> When the "boom" in chloral was at its height, a considerable number of cases were recorded showing the power of chloral to paralyze the heart, leading to fatal results, and when not going this length, the pulse became feeble and intermittent, with faintness, vomiting, shortness of breathing, and other alarming symptoms. Dr. (now Sir J.) Crichton Browne, in *The Lancet,* April 8, 1871, says: "Cases already made public prove incontestably that it (chloral) has the power of weakening the action of the heart, and even of arresting it altogether.

Brown reports an English physician, a Dr. Strange, suddenly realizing "that chloral, like several other drugs of the sedative class *operates very differently according to the amount of the dose exhibited—like digitalis, for instance—which, while in large doses paralyses, in smaller only calms and strengthens the heart's action*" (italics mine).

If he was confident that weakened chloral was very different from the non-weakened version, Dr. Patterson in all likelihood prescribed Mary Lincoln the well-known homeopathic Chloralum (homeopathic chloral hydrate) so as to *reverse* the insomniac, paralytic, heart enfeebling, pulse weakening, faintness, shortness of breath, and vomiting symptoms that addiction to conventional choral had created.

What homeopathic drugs might Dr. Patterson also have selected? Prescribing from a distance is speculative, yet cursory inspection of Mrs. Lincoln's case suggests the appropriateness of rubrics such as avarice, squanders money, ailments from grief, humiliation, mortification, ailments from fear, sleeplessness, and hysteria. These would draw up candidate remedies that include but are not limited to Clematis, Coffea, Hyoscyamus, Ignatia, Lachesis, Mercurius, Nux vomica, Opium, Pulsatilla, Sepia, and Syphilinum. What was actually recommended remains a mystery, perhaps to be revealed in future findings of homeopathic Dead Sea Scrolls.

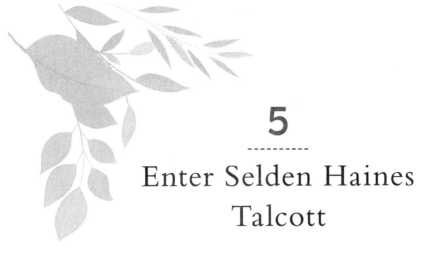

# 5

---

# Enter Selden Haines Talcott

*Innovation is seeing what everybody has seen and thinking what nobody has thought.*
BIOCHEMIST ALBERT SZENT-GYORGYI, M.D.,
NOBEL PRIZE–WINNER IN PHYSIOLOGY OR MEDICINE

Selden Talcott, perhaps the greatest psychiatrist this country has ever (not) known was born on July 7, 1842, to Jonathan Talcott and Lucy Ann Shepard in Rome, New York. His ancestry traced back to John Talcott, who came from England in 1632, and his great-grandfather Jonathan Talcott, who fought as an ensign in the Revolutionary War.

## EDUCATION AND MILITARY SERVICE

Talcott graduated from the Rome Academy, where the prizes he won in English composition and declamation foreshadowed the articulate prose and charismatic oratory for which he would later be known. In 1862 he entered Hamilton College but left the following year to enlist in Comp. K, 15th New York Volunteer Engineers and fight in the Civil War. Receiving his honorable discharge at Elmira in July 1865, he returned to Hamilton to complete his undergraduate degree in 1869. Nine years later he would obtain his Ph.D. at the same Hamilton College.

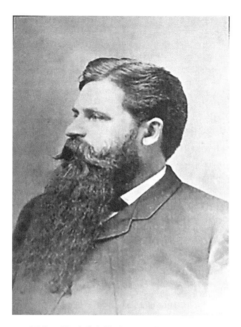

Dr. Selden Haynes Talcott, Middletown State Homeopathic Hospital
superintendent 1877-1902

Talcott began the study of medicine in 1869 under Dr. E. A. Munger of Waterville, whose daughter, Sarah, he married in 1873. Childless, the couple adopted Mrs. Talcott's sister, Ms. Cornelia Munger. In 1870 he entered New York Medical College, then known as New York Homeopathic Medical College, a school whose serious intent and commitment to scientific medicine was evident in its trustees' choice of curriculum and founding faculty appointments.

In 1860 the trustees announced "with pardonable pride . . . to the medical profession and the public" that the New York Homeopathic Medical College would be opened under the leadership of Jacob Beakley, M.D., as dean and professor of surgery, with courses of study that also included obstetrics, principles and practice of homeopathic medicine, clinical medicine, materia medica and therapeutics, chemistry and toxicology, anatomy, and physiology.[1] The study of homeopathy was unremarkably included in reputable, science-based company.

Selden Talcott graduated in 1872 as class valedictorian. His travels while studying asylum management included visits to between forty and fifty asylums in Great Britain and on the European continent. He was a member of the Masonic Order and the Concordia Leadership Council.

## HAHNEMANN DEVOTEE

A devotee of homeopathy's founder, Samuel Hahnemann, Talcott expressed heartfelt appreciation for the master in an address, "Hahnemann and His Influence upon Modern Medicine," delivered at the Homeopathic Festival in Baden, Germany, April 12, 1887. In this talk the achievements of Hahnemann that were most important to Talcott were recapitulated:[2]

1. He portrayed the true nature of disease and described it as a disturbance of vital force.
2. He enunciated the Law of Similars embodied in the doctrine *Sicut medicus utitur ut* (just as the doctor uses), a law upon which scientific medicine is inevitably based.
3. He inaugurated the plan of proving drugs upon the healthy before using them as medicines for the sick.
4. He discarded polypharmacy (the simultaneous use of multiple drugs to treat a single ailment) as unscientific.
5. He adopted the plan of using a single remedy for the safe and speedy cure of disease.
6. He made war against the popular techniques of bleeding, blistering, purging, administering emetics, and all forms of unnecessary depletion.
7. He defined medicine in a comprehensive manner.

## THE DOROTHEA DIX EFFECT

During the Civil War, Dorothea Lynde Dix served as a superintendent of Army nurses. She was a passionate American advocate on behalf of the indigent and foe of prevailing heartless treatment regimens for the mentally ill. A longtime proponent of moral treatment, Dix marshaled a vigorous and sustained program of lobbying state legislatures and the

United States Congress. In doing so she succeeded in creating the first generation of American mental asylums. At her urging the number of mental hospitals in the country, public and private, rose from 18 in 1840 to 139 in 1880, at least 10 percent of which were homeopathic. (In his book *Mental Diseases and Their Treatment,* Talcott refers to sister institutions in New York, Massachusetts, Minnesota, Michigan, California, and Missouri, but as the chapter on Talcott's disciples will show, Middletown could boast of additional offspring.[3]) Her triumph boomeranged to a large extent because in addition to mental patients the resident population of the newborn asylums began to swell with syphilitics, alcoholics, and the senile elderly.

This trend spelled doom for the movement whose values Dix championed—namely, moral care in nonmedical, small-scale (250-bed maximum) sanctuaries featuring gentle means of guidance and supervision. The new generation of asylums had a huge capacity, and the majority needs of the diverse and mushrooming population engendered cheaply constructed and culturally impoverished asylums. This invited the return of authoritarian medical oversight, underpaid and poorly qualified attendants, harsh restraints, and unnecessarily callous and experimental treatments. Dix's efforts to help a vast number of patients in effect backfired, as the humane standards she promoted could not be maintained.

## CHARITY HOSPITAL AT WARD'S ISLAND

In 1872, Dr. Talcott began the practice of his profession at Waterville, where he remained until 1875 when he received the appointment of chief of staff of the Homeopathic Hospital, Ward's Island, a charitable institution. That same year Metropolitan Hospital opened as a municipal facility on Ward's Island, housed within the Homeopathic Hospital. Its staffing, largely by the faculty of New York Homeopathic Medical College, was a great honor to the college, inaugurating what was, at that time, a rare successful relationship between a private medical school and a public hospital.[4]

Reminiscing in his 1877 resignation talk about his early days at the hospital, Talcott recalled:

*After visiting and examining the hospital building, which was the old Inebriate Asylum building of New York City, and after considering the matter as carefully as possible, I concluded to accept the position as offered by the committee of the Medical Board.*[5]

Talcott's workload and responsibilities were to accelerate. On the morning of the fourteenth of September, Talcott took charge. He writes:

*The work was new to me. The building had been put up about ten or fifteen years. At one time it was occupied by a considerable number of inebriates, but when I reached Ward's Island only about twelve cases remained under care. They occupied one ward, situated to the left of the main entrance on the first floor. The ward to the right was occupied by about fifty or sixty old soldiers, and it was called the Soldiers Home of the City of New York. . . . In addition to the soldiers and inebriates, we had an overflow of the city's insane. In two wards there were confined about one hundred and fifty patients from the city asylum.*[6]

According to Talcott the structure was in considerable disrepair. His commentary reflects the attention he would later give to the design and maintenance of Middletown State Homeopathic Hospital.

*A careful inspection revealed the necessity for numerous and varied repairs throughout the building . . . carpenter work, such as making desks, shelves, doors, etc., was accomplished by the workhouse help. The walls and ceilings of the building were freshly kalsomined [whitewashed]; bath and water-closets, steam and gas pipes were overhauled and repaired; boilers were encased in new brick jackets, and the boiler house reroofed; measurements of the entire structure were made, and every room and ward fitted up for the expected occupants.*

*Among the first of our improvements was the conversion of a large room into an amphitheater, in order that the students of the New York Homeopathic Medical College might get the benefit of clinical and surgical work performed at the institution.*

*We also sought, at the outset, to improve the dietary as far as possible, and we soon learned the value of milk and other wholesome and well-cooked foods in the care, treatment, and cure of sick people.*[7]

In short order the census of the hospital exploded. Talcott writes:

*The first year we treated four hundred and seventy-six patients, the second year three thousand and seventy-seven.*

*At the outset I acted as chief of staff of the Ward's Island Homeopathic Hospital, designed for the care of the city's poor; also, medical superintendent of the Inebriate Asylum of New York City; and, likewise, medical director of the Soldiers' Home of New York City.*[8]

Talcott's work from the fall of 1875 to the spring of 1877 in the establishment of the Ward's Island Homeopathic Hospital involved his fitting out the place with several hundred beds and, under the supervision of the medical board, directing treatment of more than three thousand patients divided among the mentally ill and the inebriated. Treatment of the mentally ill, or "insane" as they were then called, will be addressed in forthcoming chapters.

## SALOON CULTURE AND DRUNKENNESS IN NEW YORK CITY

Alcoholism was a major problem in the United States. Early Americans took a healthful dram for breakfast, whiskey was a typical lunchtime tipple, ale accompanied supper, and the day ended with a nightcap. Continuous imbibing clearly built up a tolerance, as most Americans in 1790 consumed an average of 5.8 gallons of pure alcohol a year.[9]

A measure of the challenge Talcott had signed up for is the pervasiveness of New York City's saloons, where excessive drinking was the norm. According to the census of 1790 when the population was more than 340,000, the city boasted some eight hundred taverns.[10] This worked out to one "groggery" for every 425 inhabitants.

By 1826 the count had been reduced to six hundred, but this figure takes in only legitimate taverns and fails to account for the hundreds of tippling shops and other quasi-clandestine outlets. In 1870 there were indisputably 7,071 licensed suppliers of liquor by drink in Manhattan, but again the count fails to include the proportionately vast number of illegal dives, blind tigers, needled-beer cellars, and the like which flourished mainly in the slums.[11]

## TREATING INTOXICATION

In 1890, Jean-Pierre Gallavardin published his classic, *The Homeopathic Treatment of Alcoholism,* but homeopaths had earlier gained familiarity with the problem of drunkenness and developed a concise set of remedies with which to address its various aspects. Still, the existence of a homeopathically managed inebriation asylum was then a novelty. Circulating among the hospital's six 100-bed wards would have required that Talcott be an expert keynote prescriber for the inebriates.

In so doing he would have leaned on the teachings of one of his master instructors at the New York Homeopathic Medical College, Samuel Lilienthal, a physician and a disciple of Constantine Hering, the founder of Homeopathic Medical College of Pennsylvania and Hahnemann Medical College of Philadelphia and renowned as the father of homeopathy in America. A few years after the opening of the New York Homeopathic Medical College, Lilienthal had become identified with its faculty, filling the chair of clinical medicine and that of diseases of the nervous system until his departure for San Francisco in the spring of 1887. Lilienthal was also the associate editor of the *North American Journal of Homœopathy* from 1872 until 1885.[12]

Lilienthal included inebriation-treating remedies and the subtle differentiations among them in his book *Homeopathic Therapeutics.* Talcott would thus have been well prepared to apply this knowledge to his alcoholic patients.

According to his textbook, Lilienthal recommended the following remedies for alcoholics. They are included here in detail for the benefit of my homeopathic readers. Others are invited to skim through them to note how precise homeopathic prescriptions can be. For each diagnosis there can be many possible homeopathic remedies, tailored to the individual like a custom-fitted suit of clothes, using notes about the person's nature and temperament as well as specifics of the disease itself. This is one of the secrets to homeopathy's success. Along with remedies for acute and chronic intoxication in general, and for delirium tremens, Lilienthal lists the following remedies with their indications.

**Aconitum.** When drinking wine is followed by feverish heat with tendency of blood to the head, red face and eyes, and eventual loss of reason; acute mania with frightful fancies and terror.

**Angelica atropurpurea:** Small doses will abate and prevent drunkenness; large doses (15 to 20 grs.) cause disgust for all liquors.

**Antimonium.** Gastric affections in consequence of reveling, nausea, loathing, loss of appetite, etc.; carb. veg.

**Arsenicum.** Mental derangement; anguish that drives one to and fro; fear of thieves, ghosts, and solitude, with desire to hide one's self; trembling of the limbs.

**Belladonna.** Loss of reason, delirium, visions of mice, rats, etc.; red and bloated face, tongue coated, aversion to meat, sleeplessness, stammering speech, with constant smile; dry feeling in the throat, with difficult deglutition; violent thirst, paroxysms of violent fever.

**Baryta carbonica.** Diminution of sexual desire and great weakness of the genital organs in persons addicted to the excessive use of intoxicating drinks; deficient memory; numbness of tongue and buccal cavity; tough mucus in fauces and larynx.

**Calcarea.** Delirium, visions of fire, murder, rats, and mice, where neither Belladonna or Stramonium is sufficient.

**Carbo vegetabilis.** Aching and throbbing pain in the head in consequence of a debauch; relief in the open air; nausea without desire to vomit; liquid, thin stools.

**China officinalis.** Debility of drunkards, especially when dropsy is setting in; dullness and heaviness of head as if from intoxication.

**Cimicifuga racemosa.** No disposition to talk, cross and dissatisfied;

very restless, cannot sit long in one place, sitting still makes him frantic; terrible fancies at night as if from some impending evil; tongue brownish-yellow and heavily coated; pulse quick and excited; passes only small quantities of urine; delirium tremens, with frightened look; general tremor hardly visible but apparent to the touch, with sensation to the touch of others as if cool, clammy sweat would break out.

**Coffea.** Delirium tremens; constantly running about, imagines he is not at home, with trembling of hands, with small frequent pulse; sleeplessness; overexcited; talkative; full of fear; convulsive grinding of teeth; headache after intoxication, with sensation as if a nail were sticking in the brain; worse in the open air.

**Hyoscyamus.** Epileptic convulsions in consequence of drinking; delirium tremens, with chronic spasms; averse to light and company; visions as if persecuted; sleeplessness.[13]

He would also have relied on Clemens von Boenninghausen, M.D., acclaimed earlier for finding a cure for cholera, who taught the following regarding alcoholism:

- When caused by beer instruct patient to take large quantities of Chinese tea and then as per indications Rhus toxicondendron or Nux vomica can be given.
- When caused by brandy: salt water to be given first, and later Pulsatilla to be administered.
- When caused by wine: Bitter almond [*Amygdalus amara*] to be chewed first and afterward Nux vomica to be given. And in wines containing acids, Antimonium crudum better corresponds to the indications.
- In cases where drunken person is lying with red face, staring eyes, and twitching in muscles of face: administer Opium and Belladonna in alternation after every 15 minutes, until the patient recovers, and then whatever symptoms call for.[14]

Von Boenninghausen also found that those inclined toward spirituous liquors are usually averse to drinking milk—or worse, repulsed by it—and suggested that this increased aversion should be exploited. Talcott took this advice even further at Middletown, where milk, for this and various additional reasons, became a dietary staple.

## OUTCOMES AT WARD'S ISLAND

In his 1887 address, "Hahnemann and His Influence upon Modern Medicine," delivered at the Homeopathic Festival in Baden, Germany, Talcott was able to note:

> Outside of insane asylums we find that during 1876 the death rate in the allopathic charity hospitals of New York City ranged from 8–12 percent while at the Homeopathic Hospital established on Ward's Island for the same year, the death rate was 6–14 percent.
>
> Since that year, the first after the Homoeopathic Hospital was established on Ward's Island, the death rates in all the New York City hospitals have been lighter than they were previous to the establishment of the Homoeopathic Hospital. This shows the beneficial influence of competition, as well as the beneficial effects of homeopathic treatment of disease in our public hospitals.[15]

## TALCOTT BECOMES MIDDLETOWN HOSPITAL'S SUPERINTENDENT

Talcott's success prompted an invitation to assume charge of the Middletown State Homeopathic Hospital for the insane at Middletown, New York. In accepting Dr. Talcott's resignation from the Ward's Island hospital, the medical board tendered its testimony "to the great efficiency and executive talent" he brought to bear in the administration of the hospital with "trust that success will follow him in all his future labors."

## MIDDLETOWN HOSPITAL'S
## FOUNDING AND MISSION

Born of Quaker parentage, John Stanton Gould received a thorough education, especially in physical science, and was a popular essayist and lecturer on scientific subjects. He had a farm in Columbia County, New York, and took an active part in agricultural improvement.[16] In 1866, Gould delivered a speech to the State Homeopathic Medical Society entitled *The Relation of Insanity to Bodily Disease* wherein he asserted, "It has been my purpose in this address, gentlemen, to bring before you in a clear and specific form the proofs that insanity is always a symptom of bodily disease, which it is your duty and ought to be your pleasure to cure."[17]

Gould's words ignited a resolve to create the Middletown institution. They also set the tone for the hospital's long-standing insistence on a biological foundation for its homeopathic methods.

At the next meeting of the State Homeopathic Medical Society a resolution was passed to push the New York State Legislature to construct an institution for the treatment of mental disorders along homeopathic lines. It was on April 28, 1870, that the state legislature approved a bill for the establishment of a state hospital in Middletown to use homeopathic therapy methods. The hospital opened in 1874 with sixty-nine patients. Henry Reed Stiles, M.D., founder of the American Public Health Association in New York, became the second superintendent of the hospital in 1875 and introduced strict dietary regimens. Dr. Talcott was superintendent in the hospital's glory years from 1877 to 1902, an era during which the number of buildings and patients expanded greatly, reaching more than one hundred buildings and 2,250 people in the early 1900s.[18]

## PLANNER, ADMINISTRATOR,
## AND EDUCATOR

Like Thomas Kirkbride, whom we discussed earlier, Talcott's primary concern was for the inmates, rather than the physicians. Weighing in on every aspect of how a hospital such as Middletown ought to be designed in *Mental Diseases and Their Modern Treatment*, he addresses the issue according to ten categories:

1. A suitable site for the proposed hospital.
2. The economic and durable construction of both large hospital buildings and cottages for the accommodation of various grades of patients.
3. Ventilation, heating, and lighting.
4. Protection against fire.
5. Furnishings and decorations.
6. Congregate and ward dining rooms.
7. Kitchen and bakery building.
8. Boiler house, dynamo plant [generator], and laundry.
9. Cold storage building for general supplies.
10. Outbuildings for stock of various kinds.

## A Suitable Site

In selecting the site for a hospital you should seek the moderate hilltops or sunny slopes of protecting mountains, although you should at the same time consider the difficulty of getting coal, water, and provisions to their destination without unnecessary expense. You should, if possible, locate the buildings in such a place that you may have railroad communication direct to the institution; thus the hospital will be subjected to no heavy expense for long cartage of coal or other materials. A little oversight on this point would lead, perhaps, to a subsequent expenditure of thousands of dollars per year, and without any real necessity for it.

Sites suitable for good sanitation must be attained, but to these may properly be added the inspirations of grand and stirring scenery of either the summits or the surf, and be amenable to the influence of good drainage and cultivation.[19]

## The Buildings

The buildings designed for the care of the insane should be located due north and south, or a little east of south, in order to secure throughout the *year as much sunshine as possible upon the east, south, and west sides of the buildings. After many experiments, it has been determined that hospital buildings for the insane should be not more than two stories in height. The buildings should be of moderate size, each accommodating from twenty to one hundred fifty patients. Buildings of moderate size can be furnished with light and fresh air more readily than large buildings, and patients can be more easily classified in small buildings than in large ones.*[20]

Talcott succeeded in reconciling form and function. According to a *New York Times* account from that era, in its prime the campus had temple-like chapels, huge Tudor estates for nurses, and numerous entertainment halls, as well as a "profusion of floral beauties, which constitute at once a charm and inspiration."[21]

## ADMINISTRATOR

As Jonathan Davidson writes in *A Century of Homeopaths,* "Talcott was active in various professional organizations, becoming president of the American Institute of Homeopathy and member of American Medico-Psychological Association and the New York Medico-Legal Society. He was awarded honorary membership of the Royal Academy of Medicine in Belgium. In 1889 he was appointed to the New York State Board of Medical Examiners." Emmet Dent, M.D., superintendent of the Manhattan State Hospital on Ward's Island, regarded Talcott as one of homeopathy's "most brilliant stars."[22] Talcott's skill as an administrator extended to his being for many years a director of the First National Bank and a trustee of the Middletown Savings Bank. At Middletown Hospital his leadership quickly put the facility on sound financial footing to the point where it was a showcase to the nation and the world.

## EDUCATOR

As chair of psychiatry at New York Homeopathic Medical College for sixteen years and lecturer at Hahnemann College in Philadelphia for four years, Talcott contributed to education and his textbook became a standard. His ability as a teacher directly reflected his trailblazing methods and effectiveness in treating the mentally ill.

---

### The Various Hats That Homeopaths Would Wear

Talcott's success in fields unrelated to his medical practice was not an anomaly. Flocked to by grateful patients, and often wealthier than their allopathic colleagues, homeopaths and especially superintendents of this era were held in high esteem. As prominent citizens it was not uncommon for them to also hold positions of leadership in civil and business arenas or to sit on advisory boards.

---

## TESTIMONY AT PRESIDENT GARFIELD ASSASSINATION TRIAL

Selden Talcott is remembered for his seminal *Mental Diseases and Their Modern Treatment,* the first systematic book about asylum-based homeopathic care, as well as for his remarkable inauguration of baseball into the armamentarium of psychiatry. He is also remembered for having been subpoenaed to give his expert opinion regarding a criminal case brought against Charles Guiteau, the attorney who assassinated President James Garfield. Though originally called by the defense, hoping to establish their client's innocence by virtue of his insanity, Talcott instead became convinced of Guiteau's culpability due to the man's being sane. Subpoenaed again, only this time by the prosecution, Talcott gave a discourse on the brain and insanity, after which the defense's arguments appeared feeble. Talcott's obvious knowledge and professional disport brought him praise and lasting acclaim.[23] More information about alienism (psychiatry, from the French *aliéné,* meaning "insane") appears in appendix 1, "Compendium of Madness Perspectives."

## EGALITARIAN AND
## MEDICAL FREEDOM ADVOCATE

Moneyed interests promoting disinformation and medical privatization are no recent invention. The year 1891 produced one such campaign by the wealthy designed to disenfranchise pauperized mentally ill who were eligible for care at the Middletown Hospital. Selden Talcott responded with a letter supporting a *New York Times* editorial against the measure. The following excerpts convey his outrage and compassion.

*In your issue of Feb. 19 we have read the following: "Senator Richardson has introduced a bill to exempt the Middletown Insane Asylum from the operations of the Pauper Insane bill. This institution is now on a liberal paying basis, and the fear that the pauper insane may encroach upon the confines of wealthy patients who occupy two or three rooms has led to the introduction of this bill, which on humanitarian grounds ought to be beaten."*

*The statement that the exemption from the laws of 1890, or any amendment in behalf of this hospital, is sought for because of a "fear" on the part of the friends of this institution that the pauper insane may encroach upon the "confines of wealthy patients" is untrue. No such fear exists in the minds of the friends of this hospital.*

*No private patient occupies "two or three rooms" in any of the wards of this hospital. On the contrary, no patient is allowed more than one room in a ward, and such room is often shared by one of the regular attendants or by another patient. At the present time there are 698 patients upon the census list of this hospital. Of this number but twenty-three pay more than $10 per week. The remaining 675 are either pauper or indigent patients paying low rates of board. We have nearly two hundred patients who pay from $3 to $10 per week each, and between four and five hundred who are maintained by the counties from which they come. . . . The vast majority of paying patients would be pauperized in a short time if compelled to purchase care in an expensive private institution. While we do not object to private asylums for the insane for those who wish to patronize them, we object most earnestly and strenuously to compulsory patronage of private institutions established and designed by their proprietors for the purpose of making money while* *caring for the most helpless beings on earth, to wit, persons who have been bereft of their reason.*

Lamenting the unfairness of state hospitals serving a wealthy clientele while helpless and poor mentally ill are forced into private institutions where they will be further impoverished, Talcott concludes by saying:

*There are in this State, over 1,000,000 adherents of homeopathy. As far as we have been able to learn, these patrons of our cause stand as a unit in favor of freedom of medical opinion and action.*[24]

## TRIBUTES TO SELDEN TALCOTT

Shortly after publishing *Mental Disease and Its Modern Treatment*, Selden Haines Talcott passed away on June 15, 1902. The cause was dysentery. According to Dr. Emmett Dent's memorial notice in the 1902 American Medico-Psychological Association journal:

*Dr. Talcott was modest, kind and unassuming, and a most loveable man with a great big heart, so generous and sympathetic that it embraced everyone with whom he came in contact. He was beloved by all, and as a token of tender remembrance the city closed its doors and the people attended his last honors with universal sorrow.*

*In his death, the homeopathic faith lost one of the most brilliant stars in its firmament; the country, a zealous patriot; the state, an efficient and faithful officer; and his sorrowing friends, a loyal, tender-hearted companion whose place will forever remain vacant.*[25]

# 6

# Middletown State Homeopathic Hospital's Utopian Agenda

*A map of the world that does not include Utopia is not worth even a glance, for it leaves out the one country at which humanity is always landing. And when humanity lands there it looks out, and seeing yet a better country, sets sail. Progress is the realization of utopias.*

OSCAR WILDE,
"THE SOUL OF MAN UNDER SOCIALISM"

The first American state homeopathic asylum opened its doors in 1874, sixty-six miles north of New York City, near the small village of Middletown. Officially integrated into the state health care system in 1870, the Middletown asylum had been conceived as a small bourgeois retreat with a maximal capacity of three hundred beds. It was erected in the midst of "200 acres of good, arable land, in a beautiful spot, surrounded on every side by cheerful and lovely scenery."[1]

Financed by a cooperative effort of the East Coast homeopathic community and a $150,000 appropriation from the state of New York, the facility was partly staffed with physicians from the New York Homeopathic College. The Middletown State Homeopathic Hospital was from 1877 to 1902 the domain and devoted project of Dr. Selden H. Talcott.

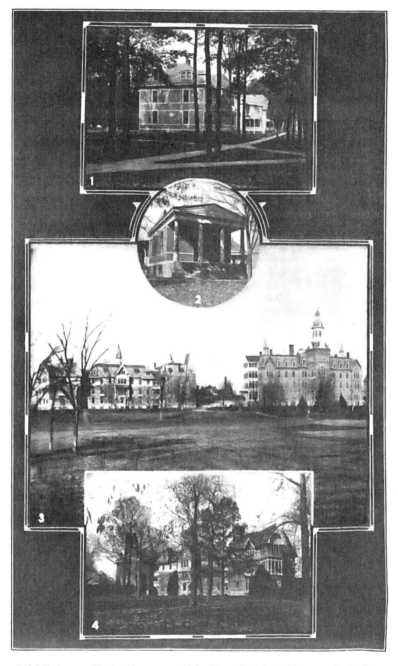

Middletown State Homeopathic Hospital 1. Cottages. 2. Bolles
Memorial Library. 3. Main Building. 4. Pavilion No. 2.

Courtesy of the American Institute of Homeopathy, from *Hospitals and
Sanatoriums of the Homoeopathic School of Medicine* (1916)

Talcott was thirty-two years old at the time and a Civil War veteran; he was aflame with ambition and idealism. Possessed of state-of-the art medical knowledge and utopian fervor, Talcott set out to:

- marry the treatment philosophy of moral treatment to Samuel Hahnemann's effective and individualized homeopathic methods in the handling of the mentally ill;
- demonstrate homeopathy's superiority to medicine of the old school;
- create a self-sustaining, budgetarily sound, full service, culturally and recreationally enriched, farm-operating hospital;
- provide occupational therapy for the mentally ill;
- provide a sanctuary for the incurable mentally ill; and
- incorporate forward-looking, scientific medical research into the hospital's mission.

Despite political impediments to his agenda, unforeseeable logistical issues, iatrogenic compromise among newly admitted patients, and continual pressure to enlarge its census mostly with paupers, Talcott's mission, especially in the early years, was successful enough to inspire ardent disciples and spawn some twenty-five satellite institutions. Before describing the Middletown Hospital's methods I'd like to review the challenges that Selden Talcott and his hospital faced.

## CHALLENGES

### The Civil War and Its Aftermath

To say that the Civil War with its economic and social upheaval, mind-numbing violence, and unprecedented carnage was traumatizing is a gross understatement. Drew Gilpin Faust, in her book *The Republic of Suffering: Death and the American Civil War,* notes how in the aftermath the populace was permeated with a grief-wracked, God-questioning, existential hangover. A tally of battleground casualties does not begin to account for it. Several factors complicated and deepened the grief:

- An afterlife belief in that era was that the dead would at some point be physically resurrected. Mutilation and dismemberment of so many of the dead sowed confusion as the notion grew unimaginable.
- Under normal conditions families expected a good death in which the dying one conveyed last words expressive of having stood by his ideals and willingly departed from the world with faith intact. The horror and seeming pointlessness of many of the battles bred cynicism among soldiers, rendering their sentiments and last words—in the unlikely event these could be heard or conveyed—uninspiring.
- The bereaved were frustrated in their attempts to learn of their sons' fates since the dead or unidentifiable pieces of them often ended up in a mass burial site, anonymous graves, or a plowed-under farm field.
- Bodies that were found intact often could not be identified. The bereaved were subjected to exhaustive, usually fruitless quests in search of fallen family members. Enormous numbers of the dead could never be located, and so closure normally associated with grieving was thwarted.

Post–Civil War suffering continued to echo from 1840 to the 1880s, when the census of hospitalized mental patients increased from 2,561 to 74,000 and the number of mental hospitals—public, private, homeopathic, and otherwise—sprouted from 18 to 139.[2] Yet the hangover's duration, and how much it instigated new or perpetuated existing mental illness among surviving veterans, their families, orphans, and widows is uncharted territory. We do note that Middletown Hospital's (thoroughly white, Anglo-Saxon) population case histories radiate anguish, grief, and religious guilt. Talcott's experience at the Homeopathic Hospital at Ward's Island treating inebriates could scarcely have prepared him for what he would face at Middletown, where his ambitious agenda for the fledgling hospital would be tested.

## Territoriality

At the time when Talcott accepted his position, homeopaths had become formidable adversaries of the orthodox medical profession. They had created their own medical societies and received sufficient support to build colleges and hospitals. However, they never constituted a majority. Outnumbered, homeopaths were pressured by a growing number of laboratory-based, medical science exponents seeking to marginalize them. Amid growing state authority, a multiplicity of health reforms, and new scientific expectations the New York state homeopaths' foray into psychiatry was infused with a quest for institutional and scientific legitimacy.[3]

Further ahead in the early 1890s, the state of New York legislated reforms designed to reconfigure care of the insane. The character of the Middletown asylum operated until then as a private hospital morphed into that of a public institution.

As a result of the State Care Act, for example, tighter control over the different state asylums and centralization of their administration was instituted. Coordinating the medical work performed at the various institutions also became a reform priority. The act not only promulgated standardization of medical training but competition between different hospitals amid an imperative of scientific productivity, all of which, rather than using homeopathic discourse, incorporated language used within the context of laboratory research.

Foreshadowing the later expansion of psychiatry outside the walls of the hospital, the Pathological Institute of the New York State Hospitals was established in 1895. Its aim was to provide "for the exhaustive study of the causes and conditions that underlie mental diseases from the standpoint of cellular biology, which is now elevated to the dignity of a special science."[4] As we shall see in chapter 11, in the hands of the Evans Research Center's* Frank C. Richardson this agenda could serve as a knife in the back of homeopathy.

It came about that New York's state mental hospitals fell under

---

*Now called the Boston University Evans Center for Interdisciplinary Biomedical Research.

the thumb of the New York State Commission in Lunacy. Tasked with coordinating pathological work conducted in the state hospitals for the insane, the Commission in Lunacy's director gained supervisory authority over all asylum laboratories, including Middletown's, allowing one member of each hospital staff to be retained by the director in the capacity of an assistant. Defending its turf, the hospital was not above hosting dignitaries or holding and publicizing gala events. The 1895 annual report of the Middletown State Homeopathic Hospital reports:

> Aside from the regular and casual visits of the members of the board of trustees, we were, last August, honored with a visit and inspection by [New York state] Governor Roswell P. Flower, who was accompanied by Colonel Judson, military secretary. On the twenty-fifth and twenty-sixth of September the State Homeopathic Medical Society met at this institution and held sessions in the Entertainment Hall. Nearly 100 physicians and their friends attended the meeting, and every city and prominent town throughout the commonwealth was duly represented. The members of the State Commission in Lunacy have made their usual visitations and inspections. The hospital has also been visited by numerous friends of patients and by the public at large. During the past summer we were favored with a visit by Dr. Louis Schepen and Dr. S. Vanden Berghe, of Ghent, Belgium. They are fellow compatriots of Dr. Jules Morel, the celebrated alienist [psychiatrist] in charge of the widely known Hospice Guislain.[5]

## Medically Compromised Clientele

At the outset of homeopathic care, then as now the physical health of one's charge is paramount. This implies the need for not only a balanced diet, fresh air, and regular exercise but also that the patient not be numbed and suppressed with conventional medications, so that homeopathy has a free and clear field of action. Then as now, a homeopath meeting a new patient hopes to operate with a clean slate. Yet in the late 1860s and early 1870s institutional psychiatrists, having concluded that a large proportion of the mentally ill was incurable, fell captive to therapeutic despair.[6] Within state mental institutions sedatives became the main drugs of choice.

Homeopaths had a rejoinder. Maintaining that the nervous system was benumbed and paralyzed by coarse, old-fashioned drugs, more benevolent medicines were offered that neither destabilized, attacked, or morbidly obstructed the patient's system. A gentler nondestructive impetus to the mind was thereby offered.

"The ordinary treatment of insane patients is calculated quite as much to injure as to benefit the patients!" Samuel Worcester declaimed at an 1872 medical society meeting.[7] Worcester, a prominent physician at the Middletown asylum, held out the example of bromide of potassium as illustrating the homeopathic advantage against injurious regular medical treatment. Worcester pointed out the effects caused by the toxic sedative, including muscular debility, dimness of sight, irregular gait, nausea, vomiting or purgation, abdominal pain, despair, and melancholy. Bromide was already being replaced in the late 1860s and early 1870s by hydrate of chloral.

Middletown homeopaths who encountered iatrogenically compromised, freshly admitted patients immediately set out to detoxify the new arrivals from their regular medicine regime. For chronic chloral poisoning, evidence of which was a patient presenting as "thin, weak, and anemic, with a poor appetite," Dr. Talcott prescribed the homeopathic Nux vomica followed by Aconite to induce sleep. We have noted that the chloral-addicted Mary Lincoln likely benefitted from a similar protocol under the care of Talcott's contemporary Richard Patterson at Bellevue Place.

## Impact of Funding

Initially patient care was supported either from patients' own estates or those of their friends, or by the counties in which they were legal residents. Under this arrangement fees from many private patients could subsidize the care of other patients supported at public expense. Passage of the State Care Act of 1890, according to which the state assumed responsibility for all mental patients, acute or chronic, making it no longer possible to receive private funding or provide private care to individual patients, ended that. Moreover, the hospital's census shifted from a mix of well-off and pauperized clients to one predominantly poor, physically broken down, and more difficult to help, as had been anticipated (see chapter 5).

## Pressure to Enlarge the Census

Over time the challenges associated with growth grew onerous. In terms both of census and its physical plant, the hospital that opened in 1874 with 69 patients expanded by the 1960s to 3,686. Individualized care and daily record keeping of a patient's progress grew less feasible. Supervision of a burgeoning population of underpaid, put-upon attendants and related help grew ever more trying. That the hospital before long would be unable to fulfill its original mission was entirely predictable.

## The Challenge of James Tyler Kent

James Tyler Kent (1849–1916) is renowned as a father of modern homeopathy in America. His massive and psychologically sophisticated guidebook published in 1897 covering physical and mental conditions and their associated homeopathics is *Repertory of the Homeopathic Materia Medica*. It was translated into several languages to provide a blueprint for all subsequent repertories, and even today is an indispensable text. Kent was a Swedenborgian Christian with an understanding of how spiritual malaise expressed itself in illness. He was adept at pinpointing the essence of a remedy picture, such as when pegging the Sulphur type of individual as a "ragged philosopher."

Kent championed the use of high-potency remedies by means of which powerful cures, especially in the arena of mental illness, could be achieved. He recommended giving a single dose of a very strong remedy, then waiting weeks or even months for its effects to unfold. I myself have used this method for more than two decades of practice and can attest to the unsurpassed power of accurately prescribed, higher potency medicines.

It is said that Kentian-style homeopathy is best suited to the setting of a private office because a very exact match between remedy and patient is demanded. This in turn requires an initial interview of two hours or even longer, not practical in a large public hospital. In addition, the high potencies of Kent's method have a certain trajectory, often taking off like a rocket—causing an immediate dramatic effect—followed by a long, drawn-out improvement. If the remedy is too strong the initial effect can be a temporary worsening, called an aggravation. Also if a second dose is given while the first one is still acting, an aggravation can ensue. All of this requires close personal supervision of the remedy effects, again not practical in a large public hospital.

An aggravation is a cathartic upsurge of past or current symptoms that for such clients could feature stormy, emotional, and behavioral release. Though such symptoms presage a condition's turnaround, aggravations would have been tumultuous, frustrating for attendants, and likely to rile neighboring inmates.

Kent's Transcendentalist precepts also confounded and irritated allopathic superintendents with whom Talcott had to rub shoulders. In certain circles an association between low-potency prescribing and so-called real medicine persists, as in France, where today nothing greater than 30 potency prescribing is permitted.

In low-potency prescribing, less dilute doses are used. Even at the lowest commonly used potency (6c) the remedy is so dilute that a physical effect of the (sometimes toxic) remedy substance is not possible. However, the effectiveness of low potencies is often confused with the effectiveness of conventional medicines, especially when the same substance is used as both conventional and homeopathic medicine, as is the case with Digitalis purpurea and other medicines. Because of the incorrect but widespread belief in Talcott's day that low-potency remedies were in the same ballpark as conventional medicines, they were more acceptable to the allopathic prescribers with whom he rubbed shoulders. Low-potency remedies blurred the distinction between homeopathy and conventional medicines, allowing homeopaths at the asylums to interact with the allopathic physicians imposed on their staff, or referring patients to them.

By the time asylum doctors such as Talcott came to appreciate Kent it was too late to change their ways. Asylum physicians found quick-acting, low-potency methods adequate to the task of calming the acute symptoms of madness. Also, unless addressing a genuinely homeopathic audience they were closed-mouthed concerning remedy potency. As we saw in the Mary Lincoln chapter, vagueness concerning dilutions had its advantages, countenancing commonality of purpose and otherwise forbidden collegiality among allopathic and homeopathic doctors.

Homeopathic asylum physicians were content for madness's singularities and underlying issues to be addressed by other components of the utopian asylum. These included the distraction of occupational therapy or farmwork, stimulation of cultural activities, contemplation of bucolic surroundings, and the compassion of well-trained nurses. Clara Barrus, both a homeopathic physician and nurse educator for fourteen years at Middletown, was preternaturally attuned to the needs of disturbed patients. So as to better instruct her charges she wrote a classic text, *Nursing the Insane.* The asylum also allowed for change to occur via the simple passage of time. Unlike today when the impetus is to "get on with it," there was less pressure then for patients to forsake the sanctuary of an asylum, especially when reentry to a frenzied, workaday world or dysfunctional family was entailed, or if the patient was powered by a mind-numbing narcotic.

## *Practicing with One Hand Tied Behind*

Little did Talcott and the other great asylum doctors know, but they could have had even better results had they known of Hahnemann's crowning achievement, a special potency (the LM or 50 millesimal potency) that could provide the advantages of both low- and high-potency prescribing. This method uses an entirely different method of dilution and potentization, resulting in remedies that are both gentle and powerful. The power of the high potencies can be attained with minimal risk of aggravation (temporary worsening of symptoms); they are as gentle as the low potencies but provide much faster improvement. Unfortunately, Hahnemann's description of this method, developed at the very end of his life, was provided in the final edition of his textbook, the *Organon,* but this edition was not published in his lifetime. In fact the manuscript was lost and rediscovered in an attic in Germany nearly a hundred years after his death, and after nearly all the homeopathic asylums had closed.[8]

At least two generations of the great homeopathic teachers that included Kent (who mastered LM prescribing) were denied earlier knowledge of a homeopathic advance that

- was gentler than the decimal or centesimal potencies;
- produced fewer aggravations than the other potencies;
- proved useful to give a patient a remedy daily, freeing homeopaths from even occasionally having to give a placebo;
- enabled "plussing" the remedy daily if given in the liquid form—this allows the medicine's potency to increase subtly, every day;
- provided a not insignificant protection: insofar as the lowest potency LM potencies remedies contain actual molecules of the original substance in defense against the denigration "Homeopathy? There is nothing in it!" is at hand and the charge that homeopathy's effect is placebo is further rebutted by pointing out that
    1. placebos are not known to produce aggravations;
    2. placebos cannot be expected to act on babies, dogs, cats, or horses as homeopathic remedies plainly do.

## HAHNEMANNIAN PRECEPTS

Instructing Talcott and bolstering his confidence that the mentally ill could be helped was the master's *Organon of the Healing Art.* Hahnemann's aphorisms about mental illness are heavy going. His teachings on mental illness may be summarized in the following paragraphs, based on aphorisms 211–29 of his masterwork.

Hahnemann discusses a primordial *miasm,* indicating a class of inherited susceptibilities from which other miasms later sprang. Designated the "itch," this is *psora.* (See in-depth discussion of psora in appendix 3.)

The physician must attend to something obvious, the strangest, least common mental or emotional feature the patient displays. This characteristic symptom provides a key clue for remedy selection.

A parallel exists between the uniqueness of the unlimited form's mental dispositions and the variety of avenues that medicinals can take so as to alter mental disposition.

Whether a condition be acute or chronic it cannot be cured other than by recourse to the Law of Similars.

Mental conditions are cured just as any other conditions are cured, according to how the remedy is researched homeopathically via provings (as explained earlier).

In a worsening mental/emotional state the physical symptoms can be seen to decline proportionately, but this is not good, as the case's one-sidedness makes it more difficult to cure. Though not a physical entity it is as though the mind is an invisible, subtle organ.

Examples are provided where the physical presentation improves as the mind deteriorates. The skill of an experienced physician is needed so that the source of the mental deterioration within physiological pathology may be located. Even so, the problem at this level is impervious to cure by surgical means.

If the breakout of madness is due to recent causes it should be treated as an acute condition. Rather than deal with an underlying existential (Psoria) issue, use familiar remedies so as to redirect the patient to his baseline state. This is adhered to in sane asylums.

The more serious forms of madness are rooted in physiology, but that is not easy to discern. Morality or lifestyle-augmenting therapies will help non-physiologically rooted cases. Such means will also *worsen* cases that are physiologically rooted (in which case accurate homeopathy is required).

Hahnemann describes a compassionate ideal according to which the mentally ill must be approached. He says that the only time coercion is justified involves the necessary administration of a homeopathic medicine that in any case is minuscule and not unpleasant tasting. How all of this works out in actual practice is best described in the text mentioned earlier, Clara Barrus's *Nursing the Insane.*

Caregivers are advised to invest themselves in a belief that the patient possesses the capacity to recover his or her reason. This means acting as if they believe and take seriously what the patient relates. As the patient is far more likely to improve in an atmosphere of tranquillity, removal of distractive amusements is recommended.

# 7

## Walking the Talk

*I know I am not a man of letters, experience is my one*
*true mistress, and I will cite her in all cases. Only through*
*experimentation can we truly know anything.*

LEONARDO DA VINCI

For a nascent republic priding itself on Christian values and morality, right up until the early part of the eighteenth century, the United States had a limited investment in the religious notion of loving thy neighbor as thyself when that neighbor was mentally afflicted. But then a compassionate zeitgeist coalesced. Fed by ardent abolitionism, Christian Science, Swedenborgianism, utopian idealism, and—above all—Quakerism, doors were flung open to welcome the moral care movement. The sanatoriums whose Mother Church was in Middletown, New York, certainly practiced moral care. But it was their employment of a medicine grounded in spirituality—homeopathy—that set them apart as special within the zeitgeist.

### TOWARD MEANINGFUL DIAGNOSES

Given his training at the Homeopathic College of New York it mattered to Talcott that prescribing for an individual on the basis of nothing other than the totality of symptoms could be reconciled with the burgeoning knowledge of anatomy and physiology. It was assumed that such prescribing reflected organic affections (maladies) such as that of the brain and that science would eventually bring those relationships to light.

The hospital reported that "an affection of the uterus, the stomach, the liver, the heart, or the lungs may, by reflex influence, tend to produce cerebral disturbance and consequent mental aberration. Hence the condition of these chief organs of the body should be carefully examined, with a view to the general treatment."[1]

Talcott classified homeopathic medicines for mental illness according to what was known of anatomy and physiology. He divided them into four groups according to their supposed localized effects (on the heart, the blood, the cerebrospinal system, or the brain).[2] I say "supposed" because a causal connection between symptoms presented by a living patient and an affected organ could often only be assumed, needing later to be established in after-the-fact fashion, postmortem by autopsy or dissection of exhumed corpses. As discussed in chapter 12 the issue of whether a mental illness is organically verifiable would eventually lead neuropsychiatry to split in two, producing the separate neurology and psychiatry professions. Insofar as "incurables" was a hospital census category, it was also considered a given that not all mentally ill patients were curable.

## MEASURING OUTCOMES

With or without diagnoses, classifying mental illnesses is context-dependent and a thankless chore. What we are measuring is unclear, so objectively assessing what Talcott, his successors, and his disciples accomplished is difficult. The thorniest problem—true in any age—involves quantifying mental illness "cures" and "improvements." There are so many variables at play. The best the asylums could do was to track unhelpful outputs such as "deaths" and "discharges." Commendably, they acknowledged, maintained records concerning, and did not cease to treat patients deemed incurable.

The following seeks to describe how the Middletown Hospital sane asylum and nearby competitor asylums operated. The reader can judge the merits of their respective inputs (the treatments).

Neighboring asylums may also be compared with regard to economic efficiency.

## MIDDLETOWN HOSPITAL'S INPUTS

Asserting a treatment principle is one thing; proving its value in action is another. How did Hahnemann's directives withstand the rigorous test of treating the insane at Middletown? I will allow Talcott his own say. The following discussion of asylum exigencies consists of excerpts from his 1902 book, *Mental Diseases and Their Modern Treatment.**

*The means we have employed at Middletown for treating the insane may be put down as follows:*
1. *Kindness and gentle discipline.*
2. *Rest as a means of physical and mental recuperation.*
3. *Bathing and massage.*
4. *Enforced protection.*
5. *Artificial feeding.*
6. *Dietetics.*
7. *Exercise, amusement, and occupation.*
8. *Moral hygiene.*
9. *Medicine (homeopathics).†*

The following sections are excerpts from more detailed explanations.

### *A General Precaution*
*In the care and treatment of the insane great caution should be exercised while the almost recovered are completing the term of convalescence. As the twilight and the dawn are the most dangerous seasons for those of suicidal tendencies, so the last days of convalescence, when the patient is feeling once*

---

*Note: there exist inconsequential organizational discrepancies between the print text and the publicly available digital version.
†Note: Talcott here sees a need to emphasize that it is homeopathic remedies that are employed, not those of conventional medicine.

*more the impulses of recovery, are oftentimes critical periods which need special attention.*

## Kindness and Gentle Discipline

*To be sure, the insane must be controlled and governed, but while the administration of discipline is at times necessarily firm and unyielding, it should in every word and action be tinctured with the essence of human benevolence. The more irresponsible the patient, the gentler and more sympathetic should be the treatment.*

## Rest in Bed

*For many years we have made constant repose in comfortable beds a prime adjuvant in the treatment and cure of insanity, and in prolonging the lives and promoting the comfort of those who are aged and feeble and unlikely to recover.*

*The victims of melancholia rise more surely from the "Slough of Despond"\* when placed in bed, and properly nourished and protected from every adverse exposure, than when they are allowed to sit up and be dressed. The victims of mania become quiet and tractable, and make better progress toward recovery in bed than anywhere else. The victims of general paresis are less liable to receive injuries, and their paroxysms of tremulous excitement subside sooner when placed in bed than when they are dressed and staggering about the ward. The victims of dementia are less filthy, and can be better cared for and made more comfortable in every way when in bed than when up and dressed, and planted in chairs along the corridors of hospital wards. Apathetic and depressed patients are not only less filthy when subjected to careful hospital treatment in bed than when up and around the ward, but they also sleep more during the twenty-four hours than they otherwise would.*

*Rest in bed does not mean neglect by nurses. On the contrary, it means increased care by specially trained nurses. The patient must be carefully and regularly looked after; his skin must be kept in good condition; his mouth must be cleansed with pure water at regular intervals; the bowels, if constipated, must be relieved by enemas of warm water; the bladder must*

---

\*The Slough of Despond is a fictional bog in the allegory *The Pilgrim's Progress* and signifies a state of extreme depression.

be emptied of its contents as often as that organ becomes filled; and baths of various kinds must be given.

## Bathing and Massage

We use baths as follows:

1. The simple towel or sponge bath, where the patient's body is laved a little at a time with alcohol and water, one part of alcohol to four or five parts of water, and then the [body] part is rubbed until dry.
2. The spray bath is used for those who are strong enough to sit up. This bath not only cleanses the skin, but stimulates by its fine and exhilarating force the subcutaneous nerves throughout the system.
3. The old-fashioned tub bath is given to those who desire it, using warm water at the outset and finishing with cold water and a brisk rubbing.

Bed patients also receive massage when necessary; and they are sometimes anointed, from head to foot, every night with cocoanut [coconut] oil, or olive oil. We use, externally, when the patient seems very much strained and exhausted, cocoanut oil, ninety-five parts, and Hypericum tincture, five parts. Hypericum is called, as you know, the "Arnica of the nerves," and this preparation is a most soothing and agreeable one. If the patient has, upon admission, recent bruises upon the body, we apply Arnica and oil in the same way. Old bruises which are dark from subcutaneous hemorrhage may be treated with Hamamelis [Hamamelis virginiana; witch hazel] and oil.

## Enforced Protection

Many of the weak and exhausted patients coming to us for treatment are quite willing to rest in bed. They are already the victims of overwork, and rest comes to them as a boon which has been desired for years. Others require to be restrained to a certain extent. This restraint, or care, or protection may be applied by a nurse who will put the patient back to bed whenever he gets up, and kindly encourage him to remain there; or, if that is insufficient, we use a body bandage. That is, a band is placed around the waist and fastened at the back with soft tapes . . . that is, tied around the bed rail.

Others are restless all over; constantly moving the legs, the arms, the *body, and the head. In such cases we apply what is known as the "protection sheet" [a camisole], which is an addition to the body bandage, and which covers the entire body, with the exception of the head and neck. When this protection sheet is carefully applied the patient cannot get out of bed, nor can he hurt himself in any way. If [the patient's] knees are chafed from motion, then he should wear drawers or a bandage may be applied, extending from the ankle to the middle of the thigh. An ordinary surgical bandage applied as if to hold a splint in place will answer the purpose.*

*Some patients are pugilistic and inclined to hurt others; or they are suicidal and inclined to mutilate themselves. We protect such cases by the use of padded mittens. Large canvas mittens are made and padded with cotton, and inside the cotton we place a smaller mitten to hold the hand. When these mittens are properly used, the patient can do but little damage to either himself or others. (The "protection sheet" was first applied at the Middletown State Hospital, over eighteen years ago, and it has been used here, as needed, ever since. It has also been introduced into many of the progressive institutions of this country.)*

*In your private practice, you may be called upon suddenly to take care of a very violent and restless case, and if you have no appliances at hand, you may make a cocoon by taking three or four common sheets, such as you will find in every house. Sew these together and roll them up like an ordinary bandage, and then apply the bandage to the entire body from the head down, just as you would bandage an arm or a leg.*

*By such a course of treatment we have had the pleasure of seeing apparently hopeless cases, after long periods of rest and nourishment, rise from sick beds and progress to genuine and substantial recoveries. After rest and care and nourishment have effected both physical and mental recuperation, then the duties and burdens of life may be gradually reassumed.*

## *Artificial Feeding*

*Insanity is a symptom not only of mental aberration, but likewise of physical depletion and cerebral exhaustion. Especially is this true with regard to the various forms, shades and degrees of melancholia and mania. We find in those suffering with mental depression, oftentimes a direct lack of desire for food, while those laboring under a stress of mental exaltation are quite* apt to neglect the inception of nourishment through inattention rather than through anorexia.

In feeding indifferent and unwilling insane patients it is always wise to begin by coaxing and persuading the sick person in the gentlest and most tactful manner to accept food voluntarily rather than to have it forced into his stomach. Many a reluctant patient will eat when properly and persistently coaxed by a skillful and judicious nurse.

The first essential in the dietetic treatment of the unwilling insane for curative purposes is the enforced administration of sufficient quantities of food, to prevent too rapid waste throughout the individual system, and to promote recuperation from losses already sustained; and likewise to increase, if possible, the capitalized resources of the human form divine [physical and spiritual strength].

The second essential is the selection of such food as will most rapidly and surely promote the rebuilding of those portions of the human temple which have been disgruntled or shattered by the effects of disease.

The third essential is the administration of the selected food in such a manner as to avoid all unnecessary shocks; to promote, in fact, easy and rapid digestion, and to favor the speedy assimilation of digested food by the tissues of the body. In our experience we have found that forced feeding may most readily be applied by the use of a soft rubber naso-stomach tube. This tube, as now used, was the invention of one of my former assistants, Dr. N. Emmons Paine, and is a modification, both in construction and use, of the soft rubber catheter of Nelaton. When this tube has been inserted through the nose, and passed on to the stomach, by a physician or skilled nurse, the food may be injected through it in required quantities by means of an ordinary rubber syringe.

## Dietetics

We come now to a consideration of the varieties of food best adapted to those depletions and exhaustions which precede and accompany mental and nervous diseases.

Owing to the restlessness and the exhaustion of the insane, and to the fact that the life forces wane rapidly, and the blood inclines to lose some of its natural fluidity, it seems to me that the diet at the outset should consist *largely of hot liquid foods, and principally of milk. The disrepute into which milk has sometimes fallen as an article of diet for either the sick or the well has arisen from the fact, to a large extent, I believe, that it has been administered cold instead of warm. Coming from the ice chest, or sipped from a glass filled with lumps of impure and death-dealing ice, and after being taken from diseased cows, it has often been a dangerous diet for even the most healthy. When milk is taken cold in large quantities it chills the weak stomach of the invalid; it curdles and forms indigestible lumps; and it ferments and brews putrescent gases in the intestines. But pure milk brought to a blood heat vents, to a very large extent, the evils of cold milk. If you have any doubt as to the purity of the milk you use, you should have it sterilized. . . .*

*In addition to milk, you may give beef tea, bean broth, and chicken, clam, oyster, and other soups. You may also give gruels made of oats, and barley, and wheat, and rice, and corn, and other cereals. You may give soups containing much cream, and flavored with such vegetables as celery, and lettuce, and tomato, and beans or peas; and you will find the various concentrated foods valuable aids to treatment.*

*An exhausted invalid should take food in moderate quantities, in order to avoid overtaxing the powers of a weakened stomach, and after each ingestion of food the organs of digestion should be allowed to do their work after which a brief period of rest may be enjoyed. But this rest should not be long continued, for if it is, then exhaustion of the patient, through lack of proper and necessary nutrition, speedily follows.*

*After many experiments, we have concluded that a weak insane person should be fed once every three hours, from 6 a.m. till 9 p.m.; and if the patient is sleepless during the night, then the food may be continued every three hours throughout the entire day and night.*

*Hot milk may, with almost absolute safety, form the daily diet and the midnight hypnotic of the mental invalid. Should such a food prove too rich in some individual case, then the milk may be diluted with lime water or with clysmic;\* or seltzer water. Should the proportion of cream in milk seem too large, then it may be reduced by skimming. Thus the amount of fat to be*

---

\*Obscure; literally refers to cleaning but likely indicated another safe diluting liquid.

*administered to a given patient may be regulated, by experience to meet the actual necessities of the case. You may also enrich milk by the addition of cream when necessary for the better nourishment of emaciated cases. The cream diet may be improved by whipping up the white of an egg with about four times its bulk off.\* Aged patients are often benefited by the use of buttermilk. In fact, all patients who have easily disordered kidneys may be almost invariably benefited by the use of fresh buttermilk.*

*While a hot liquid diet is being administered the patient may, if he craves solid food, be treated two or three times a day to a slice of toasted stale bread of such variety as he may select, that is, either white bread, or graham bread, or rye bread.*

*After a patient has, by the use of a hot liquid diet, fleshed somewhat beyond his normal weight, then he may be allowed solid food consisting largely of the various native and imported grains, together with vegetables and fruits, and a very moderate supply of meat. Rich and stimulating red meat is sometimes good for cases of melancholia, but cases of mania and general paresis should be restricted as to the eating of meat.*

*During convalescence patients may take a good deal of fat-producing food with benefit. It is better for the nervous and the excitable to take, instead of much meat, plenty of butter, and salad oil, and cod liver oil. It is always a good plan to get the patient fat as quickly as possible, but while undergoing the process, a sufficient amount of mental stimulus must be applied to keep the brain in moderately active working order while the bodily recuperation is going on. Thus the danger of dementia is averted to a considerable extent.*

*With the grain foods there may be given an abundance of fresh butter and ripened cheese, or both. Butter and cheese are simply the concentrated products of milk, and they are therefore to be reckoned among the best articles of nutrition for the human body.*

*Raw or rare cooked eggs go well with milk; and fat bacon or fat spring lamb, with baked potatoes, form excellent additions to the dietary used for the permanent recovery of the convalescent insane. Fruit is allowable in abundant quantities during convalescence.*

---

\*Obscure; may indicate introducing the more protein-dense percentage of the egg, the yolk, into the cream.

*By such a primary and secondary, or combined course of dietetics, the nervous systems of mental invalids are "renewed like the eagle's," and also by the administration of a moderate daily exercise, in conjunction with solid diet. The muscle tissues become strong again and ready for active use in the customary walks of life.*

*Those who prepare food for the use of human beings should be earnest students of psychological effects, as well as adepts in the aesthetics of cookery. The attainment of desired results in the preparation and administration of food for and to both the sick and the well is a lofty and growing ideal, and worthy of the careful study and the critical attention of everyone who is interested in the prolongation of human life, and in the preservation and continuance of health.*

*Every insane person should have at all times free access to fresh water for drinking purposes. Some persons who avoid fresh water while in their right minds will drink plenty of it when they are insane, and it seems to do them a great deal of good.*

*Stimulants are rarely needed for those suffering with insanity. The brain is in a hypersensitive condition in such cases and cannot well endure the added irritation which comes from the use of alcoholic liquors. Yet there are cases of great debility, where the stomach is too weak to retain and digest food, where champagne in small doses may be administered with beneficial effects. Sometimes brandy or whiskey may be needed to stimulate the flagging energies of a weak and failing heart. But such a resource is an infrequent necessity. When stimulants are given, only the best and purest articles should be employed.*

## *Moral Hygiene*

*Moral hygiene is just as essential in the treatment of insane persons as food is necessary for the mitigation of hunger. Moral hygiene consists in transmitting soul encouragement from the strong to the weak. Doctors and nurses should seek by kind and soothing and stirring words to inspire new spiritual energy in the lives and motives of their patients. Many a patient has been erratic and undisciplined throughout his life, and it is this lack of discipline which often brings a patient to a hospital for the insane. The establishment of mild but judicious direction on the part of those in charge of such patients is a prominent portion of their duty. Every faculty must be cultivated by means of moral hygiene; every emotion must be restrained, and every passion must be subdued, in order to enable mental invalids to possess that perfect self-control which is the loftiest attribute of sanity and strength. It is the duty of the physician and the nurse to understand one's self, to cultivate one's own powers, to be inspired by noble purposes so that the work of transmitting inspirations and disciplinary measures may be successful. This is the aim of all modern schools of psychology.*[3]

## Medicine

Lecture X of *Mental Diseases and their Modern Treatment* offers a materia medica of remedies Talcott relied on in treating melancholia, mania, paresis, dementia, and epilepsy. His approach to the madness of his day retains clinical relevance. As this section and accompanying sample of case records is lengthy and will primarily interest practitioners, the material is relegated to the appendices.

## NEARBY ALLOPATHIC COMPETITORS

Admittedly, by the 1920s the big mental hospitals, including Middletown, were much alike. Overcrowded, mismanaged, reliant on restraints, torturous treatments, and isolation, they had in effect reverted to the tendencies of the miserable, pre-moral treatment era. The condemnation they eventually received was warranted. The earlier model asylums, on the other hand, despite their architectural similarities did differ. As the following examples show, lumping together nearby facilities such as the Utica State Hospital (Utica Psychiatric Center) and the Hudson River State Hospital with the budgetarily sound and therapeutically enlightened Middletown Hospital warps the history of medicine and feeds anti-homeopathy bias.

### Hudson River State Hospital (HRSH)

Opening at almost the exact same time as Middletown and only forty-three miles away, HRSH operated from 1873 until the early 2000s. Its main building, designed by Kirkbride, has been designated a National Historic Landmark. Located on US 9 on the Poughkeepsie–Hyde Park town line, the huge facility was built at great expense on a 300-acre campus with careful attention to every detail of its design over the course of three decades.

In 1873, by which time county residents had been assured of the hospital's completion, the *New York Times* ran an editorial harshly critical of the board for not only exceeding its budget but for lavish extravagance and waste.

> The managers have entirely disregarded the law by which they were authorized to act. They have altered the plans and specifications . . . Some of the details of the extravagance of the board are amazing. For instance, the first part of the work undertaken was the construction of a reservoir, into which water was pumped from the river through an eight-inch iron pipe; from the reservoir the water was carried to the hospital by a twelve-inch iron pipe, the engine and machinery employed being on the scale of those used in supplying a neighboring city of 20,000 inhabitants. The cost of the reservoir was $100,000. Thirty thousand dollars was expended in blasting some rough rocks jutting into the reservoir, and the superintendent gave as a reason for this that, if some of the patients were missing, they might want to rake the bottom of the reservoir to find the bodies, and with this the rocks would interfere . . . The floors are laid in yellow Southern pine, the most expensive of the flooring, fitted and cut in a way greatly to enhance the cost. The heating is arranged on a scale that, with only 150 patients, ten tons (9 tonnes) of coal per day is consumed. The mention of these items sufficiently explains the disappearance of $1,200,000 of the people's money.

Despite efforts to stop the project, the legislature continued to appropriate funds, even amid further revelations of corruption. Construction continued until 1895, when the money pipeline finally froze. The hospital's original plan was still not complete, and never would be.[4]

As at Middletown, HRSH offered moral therapy, a stimulating environment, vocational training, art, music, and congregate activity. Nursing formed the backbone of the care. In place of homeopathy the hospital's means of treatment did not go beyond hydrotherapy, and the medications: paraldehyde, bromide, chloral, luminal, and various tonics.[5] Apart from being a money pit, which Middletown Hospital was not, the two facilities differed only in Middletown's offering homeopathy. Hudson River's non-homeopathic treatment outcomes could have served as an ideal control when compared to Middletown's outcomes had a study of homeopathy then been in the offing.

In copycat fashion Hudson River State Hospital jumped on the baseball bandwagon that Middletown had pioneered as a diversion for its patients. It seems right and fitting that when the teams played each other in 1891, the great Middletown asylum's nine prevailed over the HRSH team by a score of eight to seven.

## Utica State Hospital

One hundred and twenty miles from Middletown Hospital, the New York State Lunatic Asylum, later named the Utica State Hospital, and known locally as Old Main, was built in 1843. Pre-dating Middletown, it was the first publicly funded institution in New York State to treat the mentally ill and so considered for that time a prototypical effort to provide mental health care in an institutional setting. Patients were first admitted in 1843, although its construction had not yet been completed.[6]

The facility's first superintendent, Dr. Amariah Brigham, published the *American Journal of Insanity* at the asylum in 1844. It was the first journal of its kind published in English and helped grow Utica's reputation as a center of psychiatry.

Brigham was a proponent of labor as the most essential of our curative means. He thus encouraged patients to engage in tasks such as gardening, handicrafts, needlework, and carpentry. Brigham also introduced an annual fair at the hospital to display and sell items created by the patients. Some of the asylum inmates also printed a newsletter.[7]

Brigham was less imaginative than Talcott, whose subtle understanding of enforced restraint and use of the camisole (straitjacket) I have touched on. As an alternative to using patient-restraining chains, the Utica director practiced a form of moral care that resorted to an infamous device akin to confinement pens utilized at St. Peter's Hospital, Bristol, England in the early 1800s.[8]

Introduced in 1846, the Utica Crib, as it came to be called, was an ordinary bed with a thick mattress on the bottom, slats on the sides, and a hinged top that could be locked from the outside. It was eighteen-inches deep, eight-feet long, and three-feet wide. Enclosed within its confines the patient could barely move. The expression "to become unhinged" may stem from a recognition of a Utica patient's state of mind upon being freed from it. Doctors and staff used the horrifying cage to calm, break the spirit of, and punish patients.

Though unaffiliated with the Utica State Hospital, in 1901 a nascent New York State League baseball team from Utica, with a nod to the hospital, named itself "The Pent-Ups."

# 8

## Play Ball! The Innovation of Baseball Therapy

*You see, you spend a good piece of your life gripping a baseball, and in the end it turns out that it was the other way around all the time.*

JIM BOUTON, *BALL FOUR*

America has always enjoyed watching a group of skilled players club, hurl, and snag a ball in competition, and baseball has been a favorite since English colonists brought it over amid their baggage. Always fun, entertaining, challenging, and good exercise, it wasn't until the late 1800s that anyone conceived of baseball's value as therapy.

### THE MARVELOUS ASYLUMS TEAM

I am grateful to Bob Mayer, a longtime member of the Society for American Baseball Research (SABR), for generously allowing me access to his extensive and unique baseball memorabilia archive and granting permission for use of text from his article "The Asylum Base Ball Club: Middletown's Crack Semi-Pro Team 1888–94," on which this section is based.

Middletown, New York, was a rural community of about thirteen thousand people in 1888. A part of Orange County, it lies along one of the main routes from New York City to the Catskill Mountains, which were becoming a major recreation area for New York residents at the end of the nineteenth century. The village was home to the Orange County Brewery, several foundries, a hat factory, a local bottling plant, and several popular hotels. It was also a hub for the New York & Lake Erie Railroad, as well as the New York, Ontario & Western Railway, and had been the home of the Orange County Fair, a popular yearly event since the early 1880s.

For New Yorkers, 1888 may be remembered as the year of the great blizzard, which dropped three-and-a-half feet of snow and paralyzed the Northeast for days. Middletown residents were then likely dreaming of springtime when their local baseball team, the Wallkills, could take the field. Formed in 1866 by prominent town citizens, the Wallkills had ever since been competing against other town and barnstorming teams. The year 1888 was a milestone in other ways as well, being the year that the village of Middletown became a city and when the mental hospital's Asylum Base Ball Club was organized.

During Selden Talcott's tenure as head of his utopian institution the patient census expanded from 228 to more than 1,200. The nearly self-sufficient hospital possessed its own farm, power station, laundry, and trolley stop. Amid this bounty Talcott's vision widened to encompass amusements and recreation in any way supportive of patient well-being. Enthusiastically he garnered an array of cultural and sports-related activities under the asylum's umbrella. According to Bob Mayer,

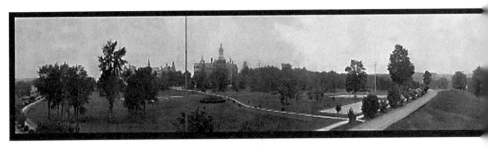

The entrance to the hospital grounds in 1906, with the main building in the background. The original ball field can be seen to the left of the road leading to the main building.
Courtesy of Bob Mayer

playing baseball is recorded to have been encouraged for the mentally ill in New England as early as 1838, so Talcott's having a baseball field cleared proximal to the main building is not surprising.

As the Middletown asylum's patient newspaper, *The Conglomerate,* tells it, one day in 1888, Talcott witnessed a ball game on the grounds among the attendants and patients. While sitting there, he became impressed with how engrossed in the game his patients became. Afterward he called a meeting of his staff to obtain support for forming a baseball club and succeeded. Dr. D. H. Arthur was appointed president, and Hospital Supervisor Wilbur Cook, who happened to have had previous baseball experience, agreed to be manager. That first year the team played seven games, winning four, losing two, and tying one. Three of these games were against the Wallkills Base Ball Club, a local amateur team that included players who would go on to careers in the major leagues.

Poaching some of the best local players (several from the Wallkills) and others he knew from out-of-town teams, Cook soon built his team into a local powerhouse.

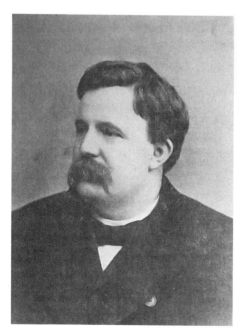

**Manager of the Asylum Base Ball Club**
Courtesy of Bob Mayer

To ensure that the games would be exciting to both the patients and the large crowds assembling from neighboring towns, Talcott sought out the most competitive teams for the Asylums to play. He also persuaded the Asylum trustees to guarantee his team adequate equipment, uniforms, and even travel expenses. To defray the cost, the public was charged an admission fee of twenty-five cents at most home games, with a good number of season tickets being sold to ardent fans.

Not only did Talcott rarely miss a game, but he proved a savvy motivator and salesman, too. It was the superintendent's practice to award a "fiver" (five dollars cash, not a "high five") to any home team player who bashed a home run during a game. A financial hit to the doctor, the practice was a hit with the crowd, who egged the players on with a "go for the fiver" chant whenever a player reached third base. On game days not only were the patients escorted to the field to watch their team play, but many of those too ill to come outside were coaxed to pavilion windows from which perches they could root for their heroes.

The 1889 Annual Report of the Middletown State Homeopathic Hospital for the Insane to the State Commission in Lunacy reflects baseball's positive impact on the patients.

The beneficial effect of the national game upon those whose minds have been depressed or disturbed is very marked. The patients in whom it had hitherto been impossible to arouse a healthy interest in anything seemed to awaken and become brighter at the crack of the sharp base hit. Even demented patients were eager watchers of the game. No game has ever excited such universal interest on the part of the inmates of the asylum. Even those who were very sick would insist upon being propped up by pillows so that they could look out the windows and watch a game while it was in progress.

In 1889, the Asylum team's first full year, the team won eleven games, lost three, and tied one. The fourth player from the left is Fisher Launt. Two players to his right is John C. Degnan, and the second player from the right is Pat McGreevy. These players were previously on the Wallkill Base Ball Club and (unless they at some point went crazy) were never Middletown Hospital residents.

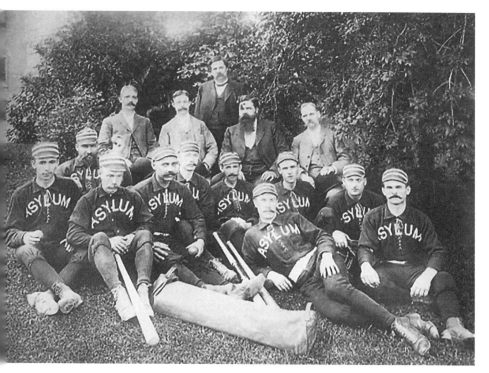

**The 1889 Asylum Base Ball Club**
Courtesy of Bob Mayer

The Asylum club was not only playing other teams from Orange County, but also attracting some fine teams from New York City, Brooklyn, and New Jersey. One team that made the journey to Middletown was the Actors' Amateur Athletic Association of America, better known as the 5As.

The teams split two games in 1889, and the Asylums won another from the 5As in 1890. The Asylum team had a great year in 1890, winning twenty-one games and losing only four. But the best was still to come.

DeWolf Hopper, one of the more famous of the players, was an actor and matinee idol noted for his performances in Gilbert & Sullivan operas. His several wives included actress Elda Furry, who is best known as Hollywood columnist Hedda Hopper. He is most famous, however, for being the first to recite in public,

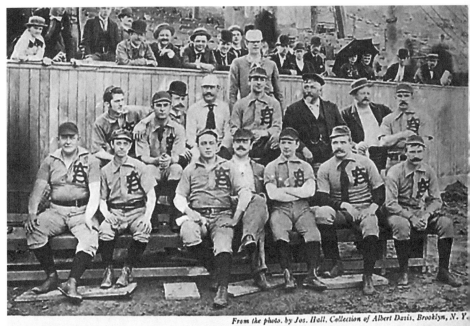

*From the photo. by Jos. Hall. Collection of Albert Davis. Brooklyn, N. Y.*

THE ACTORS' TEAM THAT PLAYED THE NEW YORK PRESS CLUB IN 1889

Mr. Hopper stands at rear, Francis Wilson, seated, below him, and below the latter is Wilton Lackaye at left, James T. Powers at right

**The 5As Base Ball Team 1889**
Courtesy of Bob Mayer

on August 14, 1888, Ernest Lawrence Thayer's poem, "Casey at the Bat."

In 1892 the Asylum team beat virtually all comers. The team had wins against strong New York City teams including the Gorhams and Alphas. They also defeated the Allertons of New Jersey and the Black Professional Cuban Giants. Only the New York Giants with Hall of Fame players Buck Ewing, Mickey Welch, Jim O'Rourke, and Amos Rusie defeated them. The team won twenty-two games and lost only two. The Giants squeaked out 2–1 and 6–5 (ten innings) wins.

Season record: won twenty-two, lost two (both losses were against the National League New York Giants).

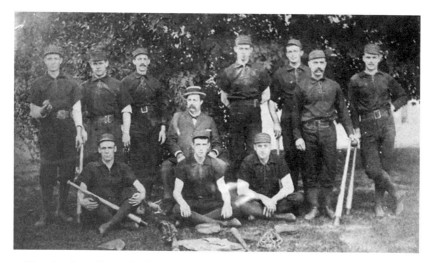

The Asylum Base Ball Club in 1891, together with the old Wallkills
(Degnan, McGreevy, and Launt) and Chris Genegal (standing third
from right), who joined in 1889, formed the core of the team
for several more great years. Additions included Tommy Murray
(standing second from left) from the New York Arlingtons, John Lawlor
CF standing far right, and Jack Dooley 1B sitting in front of W. Cook.
This 1891 team won thirteen and lost seven.

Courtesy of Bob Mayer

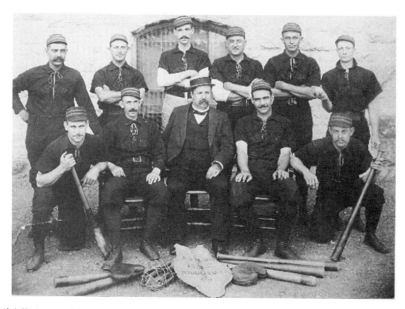

Middletown State Homeopathic Hospital Base Ball Team 1892 (partial)

Courtesy of Bob Mayer

The hospital's 1892 Annual Report to Albany commends baseball yet again:

After several years of experiment, our medical superintendent claims that baseball as a craze displaces other crazes and helps to relieve the mind of its troubles and delusions. There is ample evidence for this belief, and any one at all acquainted with the insane has only to attend a ball game on the asylum grounds, or go through the wards on the day of a game to feel its full force. . . . On the day of a ball game everybody is astir. A thrill of absorbing attention of what is going on, all due to the healthy stimulus and the fascinating character of the national pastime.

One of the more interesting teams played during the 1894 season was the Minneconji Indians team from the Minneconji Reservation of Missouri. On July 9 the Asylums faced a fearsome group of players with this line-up:

| | |
|---|---|
| Running Antelope | C |
| Killing Horse | P |
| Two Belly | 1B |
| Man Who Sleeps | 2B |
| Shooting Star | 3B |
| Running Fast | SS |
| Buffalo That Bellows | RF |
| Frisking Elk | CF |
| Bounding Pony | RF |
| Bull Head | Captain |

This team of Native Americans was managed by the theatrical trio of Miaco, Ball, and Blum, who promoted the barnstorming outfit all over the country. The team played rather well, although the Asylums triumphed twenty to ten. As expected from the era, the papers had some fun with the players' names: "The Man Who Sleeps woke up suddenly and made a two-bagger . . ." and "Running Antelope ambled to first. . . ."

## MIDDLETOWN'S HALL OF FAMER

Destined for enshrinement in baseball's Hall of Fame was (Happy) Jack Chesbro, who in 1894 at the age of nineteen first arrived at Middletown Hospital to work as an attendant. Chesbro would become a starting pitcher for the New York American League franchise—a team variously nicknamed by the press as Highlanders, Hilltoppers, and even Yankees. In 1904, Jack won forty-one games and pitched forty-eight complete games, still top totals for seasons after 1893.

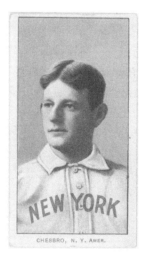

Jack Chesbro
baseball card,
1901-1911

## THE BENIGN MADNESS OF
## DEEP ABSORPTION

We chill out at the ballpark, but there's so much more to it. A baseball game is relatable due to the vivid individuality of its players, their skills, and also their quirks, bumblings, and heroic acts. It is absorbing for spectatorship demands our attention. Within the vast panorama of the field, visual acuity is required just so that the tiny pitched or batted ball's movement can be tracked.

The most casual fan may record a game's every play in a score sheet; memorize batting averages, on-base percentages, home runs, and runs batted in statistics; or retain the indelible image of a player's batting stance and mannerisms. Decades later the information is retrieved, critical games dissected and debated. For example, Boston Red Sox manager Johnson "shoulda nevah took Willoughby outa the seventh game of the 1975 World Series against the Reds!"

## WELLNESS AND RELATABILITY

Baseball is relatable for ushering its audience into an alternative universe, a locale in which individual membership and personal relevance are palpable. Uniquely, the game does not follow a clock. As in life, time in baseball registers only concluded events, "outs" made, three of which compose half an inning. Just as with human life span a game's length can vary, its duration ranging from how long it takes to complete five innings (a rain-shortened game), eight and a half or nine innings (the usual length), or, in the event of a tie after nine innings, additional innings. Games have been played that dragged on for more than a day. Provided that outs are not made, a contest could go on forever.

Everyday life is often humdrum. A baseball game, too, is largely uneventful. Much of the time little seems to occur other than the players fidgeting, chewing, spitting, posing, squatting, stretching, or yawning. But then all at once players on the field tense with alertness, ready with the smack of a ball to spring into action. The game's pokiness encourages gabbing among spectators but also allows for spirited bantering with players within shouting distance.

Demands placed on professional players for the most part appear so ordinary that anyone could do them: amble over to a popped-up fly ball, camp under and catch it; corral a grounder and then toss the ball ninety feet to first base; trot around the bases after a home run. To our relief what appears to be embarrassing within baseball is rendered endurable: the ignominy of swishing, swinging, and not making even the slightest contact with a pitched ball is ruefully accepted. The most skillful hitters fail to reach base two-thirds of the time. Making their out they do little more than shrug when ambling back to the dugout.

The game is often lunch-pail routine. As in life, circumstance dictates the need for an occasional out-of-the-norm act, a stepping up of one's game. It may be the star slugger who is summoned. It can just as easily be a lowly utility player. *Some* player must make the brilliant catch, the timely hit; or execute the heads up run-down play rescuing the beleaguered pitcher from further clobbering, and on which the outcome of the game depends.

Baseball's honoring of moral equivalence is evident in ground rules allowing foul lines to be traversable. A ball batted into foul territory remains playable; a runner churning around third base on his way home can meander over to the out of play side of the foul line; the outfielder making a brilliant outfield catch robbing the batter of a home run may tumble completely out of the playing field; though not a participant, the fan sitting in the stands who interferes with a playable ball can critically alter a game's outcome (see Steve Bartman and the famous billy goat curse, related to a malodorous goat whose offended owner allegedly cursed the Cubs team).

## RELATEDNESS AND VILLAINY

We can all relate to a villain. Nodding along, baseball enables crime to pay. Theft, as in base-stealing, is laudable. The art of pitching involves nothing so much as deceiving the batter and may include physical doctoring of the pitched ball to make it veer unpredictably. Base runners must remain alert to the hidden ball trick. The innocently trusting get tagged out. Stealing coded signs from the coaches or between the catcher and the pitcher (though not with the aid of video cameras) is a time-honored if not entirely respected practice.

With finagling, the not-so-kosher is made kosher. Though objectively every pitch is either a strike or a ball, depending on his disposition that day or his unofficial relationship with the pitcher an umpire can expand or contract the strike zone during a game. As is true elsewhere in life, when encountering unfairness one is often better served by adjusting than by griping.

## CRAZINESS AND QUIRKINESS

To be crazy is fairly normal within baseball, the word *fan* itself being short for "fanatic." One of the most famous announcer cries, which followed the final 1951 game between the Dodgers and the Giants (Bobby Thompson's homer being called "the shot heard round the world") was Russ Hodges' exuberant "The Giants win the pennant! They're going crazy!" The game abounds with beloved and zany characters. Some, such as Jimmy Piersall, who battled bipolar disorder, were prone to genuine mental disturbance. Similar to Belgium's system of family patronage in Geel, baseball's tolerance of eccentricity provides its Piersalls a generally safe haven. How crazy is it that in baseball but no other sport is a team's manager or coach, usually a pudgy, middle-aged and cranky taskmaster, obliged to stuff his ungainly torso into a completely unnecessary athletic uniform?

## A FIELD AT ONE WITH ITS ENVIRONMENT

Historically, baseball parks and stadiums are designed to be in harmony with their environment, whether that be rural or urban. This accounts for the charming quirkiness of stadiums such as Fenway Park and Wrigley Field. To soothing effect, the field adjacent to the main building at Middletown Hospital blended with the bucolic neighboring countryside.

## EMBRACING THE EMOTIONS

In their mania fans can lose their minds. For the true believer, especially the masochistic aficionado of a longtime losing team, baseball bursts with tragedy, gloom, disappointment, and despair, making the team's rare breakthrough triumph all the more glorious.

Fans of a losing team must endure long-term suffering, but players can suffer right along with them. Pitcher Ralph Branca never got over giving up the immortal Bobby Thomson ninth-inning home run, an epic tragedy for the Dodgers in a 1951 play-off against the Giants.

In robust fashion players are admired, reviled, and often hilari-
ously nicknamed for their physiques, demeanor, predilections, names,
nationality, and accomplishments. One of the greatest players, a raging
alcoholic who played like a mad dog, was ironically called the Georgia
Peach (Ty Cobb). Babe Ruth was known as the Sultan of Swat. Among
my favorites: Bill (the Spaceman) Lee, (Oil Can) Dennis Boyd, Leo
(the Lip) Durocher, George (Piano Legs) Gore, Stan (the Man) Musial,
Lawrence (Yogi) Berra, Al (the Mad Hungarian) Hrabosky, Mark (the
Bird) Fidrych, Fred (Bonehead) Merckle; and the great Jewish relief
pitcher and all-time "saves" record holder, Mordechai (the Messiah)
Nathanson. I made up that last one. He has yet to come.

Umpires—God-like father figures and supposedly impartial
arbiters—are typically held by spectators to be blind. Up to a point they
tolerate being argued with, raged at, and having dirt kicked in their
general direction. An apoplectic team manager having such a tantrum
will more likely be repaid with a boot out of the game than a call reversal. Still, the fuss makes for wondrous theater.

## ODD DUCKS

One way or another we are all odd ducks, a truth that baseball does
honor. Though on the whole professional baseball players are wondrous athletes and look the part, space exists for odd ducks: puny,
overweight, or middle-aged specialists, or the rare player with a lone,
situation-specific skill. Veteran catcher Smoky Burgess of the Pittsburgh
Pirates was one, overweight and old in baseball years, his extended tenure ensured by his bankable pinch-hitting ability. Lanky Yankee pitcher
Ryne Duren was so nearsighted as to be legally blind, making him
one of the worst hitters in baseball history. His roster spot was secure
because he could hurl a ball almost one hundred miles an hour, terrifying batters who encountered him.

A track and field star devoid of baseball skill can make a team as
a pinch runner. A rare brand of pitcher is the knuckleballer, a generally nonathletic artist whose unsettling, spin-less throw mystifies not
just the batter but the catcher and the pitcher himself. Teams find it

advantageous to carry a "sparkplug," a feisty, sometimes heady infielder with a big mouth willing to taunt an umpire, incite his teammates, rile the opposition, or create havoc just for the hell of it. He evolves into a coach or manager.

## WHO, ME A BONEHEAD?

We hoot at the bonehead but also cringe, since there but for the grace of God go I. Ah well, laughter is the best medicine and so we revel in Marvelous Marv Throneberry of the original Mets hitting a triple and somehow managing to sidestep not just one, but two bases. Guilty pleasures include 1908's immortal bonehead play when Giants player Fred Merkle's failure to advance to second base on what should have been a game-winning hit led instead to a force-out at second, tying a game. The Cubs later won the makeup contest, beating the Giants by one game to win the National League pennant. We relish the saga of a group-effort blunder concocted by the hapless 1926 Brooklyn Dodgers, which incredibly culminated with three teammates simultaneously perched atop third base.

## EXISTENTIALIST HUMOR

Unprepossessing as a baseball may be, the lone ball happening to be in play possesses a magical property. It is *live*. In one historic game puzzler (I believe the fabulous original Mets were involved), a throw from the outfield went astray and bounced into the dugout of one of the teams. So as to retrieve the ball and possibly tag out the runner who may have missed home plate, the catcher, pursued by the umpire, hustled into the dugout and found, to his astonishment, that the ball had wangled its way into the ball bag!

An existential question arose: Which of the balls is live? After a tense interval the catcher, ball in hand, again pursued by the umpire burst forth from the dugout in search of the runner. Only the runner by now had disappeared. The already flustered umpire declared him safe at home. No one has ever disclosed how the magically live ball came to be differentiated from the other balls in the bag. The mystery is absorbing, but also funny. Maybe you had to be there.

## SUPERSTITIOUS

Catty-corner across from obsessive-compulsive disorder lives a more socially acceptable neighbor, superstition. More than in any other sport, the prevalence of ritualistic behavior in baseball fosters connection with the fan. Baseball's relatable rituals include:

- not talking about a no-hitter or perfect game while the game is in progress;
- players eating the same exact meal before every game;
- hopping over the foul line when approaching it;
- engaging in a repetitive batting-stance ritual;
- flipping a rally hat inside out to spark a rally (fans participate in this as well);
- avoiding a pitcher alone on the day of his star;
- pointing skyward after hitting a home run;
- constantly adjusting batting gloves while in the batter's box awaiting a pitch; and
- wearing only lucky socks during a winning streak, and always using a particular lucky bat or gloves.

## LIFTING A CURSE

Similar to the notion of having been born under a bad sign lives a more delusional belief, that of being cursed. A famous example of this is the curse of the bambino, referring to the inability of the Boston Red Sox to win a World Series after the team's owner sold the New York Yankees their star player, Babe Ruth, for a piddling sum. The Babe, as it turned out, became the greatest player in the history of baseball, thus winning reference to the infant Christ. Wearying of the lamentations of woebegone Red Sox fans, the gods of homeopathy in 2004 called a halt. Homeopathy was invoked so that the Red Sox could miraculously come from behind to win a playoff game against the Yankees and then in the World Series, rout the National League's St. Louis Cardinals to end the curse.

Rather than being mystical the infamous curse represented an entrenched fear and an associated managerial rigidity. Homeopaths routinely implicate similar inflexibilities as key factors underlying their patients' disease states. But "remedy states" need not be cured by homeopathic remedies alone. The homeopathic practice of "prescribing the symptom" can also do the trick.

The fear underlying the curse of the bambino was that team management might once again commit an error as egregious as giving away the great bambino. The pursuant rigidity was: beware of making any baseball trades even remotely suggestive of this possibility. When installed as a core front office rule, a fear such as this delimits flexibility and creativity, and disadvantages the team with respect to other teams in the trading marketplace.

A shibboleth exists in baseball that the value of even a handful of good players cannot equate that of a single great player, the ostensible reason being that truly great players are irreplaceable while many even very good players are readily exchanged for others of equal value. Avoidance of such trade would be in keeping with the fear and associated rigidity of the bambino curse. But just as homeopathy teaches that like cures like, the recommended solution involves a reengagement with the original error, via a microdosage of the mistake. Frightening though it seems, directly facing the demon trumps doing nothing.

Red Sox shortstop Nomar Garciaparra was anointed the greatest Red Sox player since Ted Williams by no less a luminary than Ted Williams himself. Yet in 2004, General Manager Theo Epstein, whispered to by the homeopathic gods in his sleep, opted to trade the inimical and irreplaceable Garciaparra for three talented but lesser lights: outfielder Dave Roberts and infielders Orlando Cabrera and Doug Mientkiewicz. On the day the trade was announced talk show radio hosts went berserk and the trade was denounced in the newspapers as another Babe Ruth giveaway. Yet Epstein's decision inexplicably propelled the team to a peak performance, thereby allegedly lifting the curse. As told in

Harvard psychiatrist Eric Leskowitz's 2010 book (also made into a film) *The Joy of Sox,* the Red Sox's incredible triumph rocketed the spirits and mental equilibrium of countless New Englanders. Somewhere, Selden Talcott is smiling.

In the National Football League in 2021, yet another New England team seems to have incurred a curse. With their great quarterback Tom Brady, an uncontested free agent parting ways with their Patriots, fans gaped in astonishment as their longtime hero promptly won a Superbowl for his new team, the Tampa Bay Buccaneers. A woeful cry for relief has been raised. Will the gods of homeopathy again respond?

## THE HEALING POWER OF RITUAL

Extending the notion that rituals are relatable, we have a sublime proposition from Hannah M. G. Shapero. Her article "The Diamond Way: Baseball as an Esoteric Ritual" makes the case that attendance at a baseball game provides the spiritually elevating experience of a sacrament. I offer only the beginning of her exegesis.

It is the vernal equinox and the ritual has begun. The participants enter into the sacred quadrant and take their stations at geometrically significant places. They are all men, dressed in pure white garb, marked with colorful esoteric symbols. They hold ritual implements in their hands. Four more men arrive; they are dressed in dark blue. Like concelebrating priests, they confer on the details of the liturgy. Then they too take their places.

A sacred hymn is intoned, and after that come the opening words of the ceremony: "PLAY BALL!"

We need look no further than the local baseball diamond to find high ritual. There is no need to hanker after secret Masonic rites in closed halls or occult workings in incense-filled chambers. Wherever baseball is played, a true ritual goes on, as exoteric as daylight, as powerful as spring.

Far more than other sports, baseball shows an esoteric structure. The game is played on a geomantically perfect square. Each base stands at what would be the quarters in Western esoteric ritual. These four bases also stand for the four elements, though attributions are variable: Home plate, with its coating of dust, seems to be Earth, while third base is traditionally referred to as the "hot corner," signifying Fire. In the center is the pitcher's mound, a circle in the middle of the square mandala, which speaks to us of the fifth element of Spirit, or the center point of wholeness.[1]

## IN THE SPIRIT OF SELDEN TALCOTT

In 2017 a gerontology research paper titled "Influence of Watching Professional Baseball on Japanese Elders' Affect and Subjective Happiness" was published. The self-evidence of its conclusion would have made Selden Talcott beam, but the scientist in him would have appreciated the study's rigorous design. Below is the paper's abstract.

**Objective:** To determine the effects of watching a professional baseball game on the affect and subjective happiness of elders without a specific team to support.

**Method:** Elderly Japanese (n = 16) were instructed to watch baseball games at a ballpark. They answered a questionnaire several weeks before (baseline) and on the day of the game, before and after watching the game. Participants' affect and happiness were assessed using the General Affect Scale and Subjective Happiness Scale, respectively.

**Results:** Calmness had a tendency to increase from baseline to before watching the game (p = .052). Furthermore, subjective happiness significantly increased after watching the game, compared with baseline ($p$ = .017).

**Discussion:** Visiting a ballpark to watch a professional baseball game increased elders' subjective happiness after they had finished watching it.[2]

The truth of an adage coined by the sage Yogi Berra is affirmed: "You can observe a lot by just watching."

# 9

## Genius Physician
## and Nurse-Educator
## Clara Barrus

*You must never so much think as whether you like it or
not, whether it is bearable or not; you must never think of
anything except the need and how to meet it.*

CLARA BARTON

Before we can talk about Clara Barrus, a heroine in her own right,
we must acknowledge her predecessor named Clara. Beloved and
famous, educator and nurse possessed of a warrior spirit: that would
describe Clara Barton. Known as the Angel of the Battlefield for repeatedly risking her life to bring supplies and support to soldiers in the field
during the Civil War, Barton's life set a high-bar example for how to
overcome the inequalities of society while demonstrating to men the
infinite capability of women. An experience early on when she built a
school providing free education for hundreds of youngsters, but then on
sexist grounds was denied the run of it, inflamed Barton's determination. In 1881, at age fifty-nine, Barton founded the American Red Cross
and led that formidable organization for the next twenty-three years.

Playing yin to Barton's yang was another, lesser known "Clara Bar"
educator and health care warrior. Whereas Clara Barton was afire to
meet the needs of Civil War soldiers and their families, Clara Barrus's

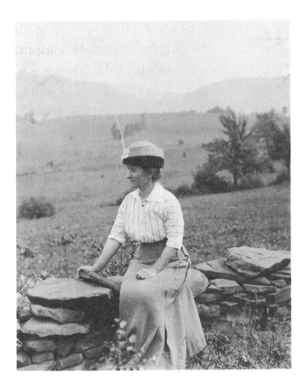

Dr. Clara Barrus

flame burned with equal intensity on behalf of the needs of an equally suffering but more hidden population—the mentally ill.

Born in Port Byron, New York, in 1864, Clara Barrus studied medicine at Boston University and received her Doctor of Medicine degree in 1888. For several years she was in private practice in Utica, New York, but in 1893 she became an assistant physician under Selden Talcott at the Middletown Hospital, where she exercised an abiding interest in nursing. She also served as professor of psychiatry at Women's College of New York City, which had been founded by renowned womens' rights champion and homeopathic physician Clemence Sophia Harned Lozier.

Dr, Lozier was a cousin of Carroll Dunham, president of the American Institute of Homeopathy and of the World's Homeopathic Convention of 1876. After graduating from university with high honors in 1853, she opened her practice in New York, where she commenced giving popular weekly health talks out of which an idea germinated to form a medical college for women. By 1863 she had secured passage of an act by the legislature granting the charter for a medical college for women upon which the New York Medical College was opened.[1]

As caretakers of the family health, women had in many communities assumed the role of homeopathic lay prescribers and become professionals as well. By 1900 approximately 12 percent of homeopathic physicians were women,[2] and undoubtedly many of them were students of Clara Barrus. Members of the women's suffrage movement were often homeopathic physicians, patients, or advocates, such as homeopath Elizabeth Cady Stanton[3] and Dr. Susan Edson, a graduate of the Cleveland Homeopathic College, who served as personal physician to President James Garfield.[4] In Ohio in 1871, the Cleveland Homeopathic Medical College was one of the first coeducational medical institutions of any kind in the country. All indications were that there was an ongoing need for women's medical education, and Clara Barrus was supremely qualified to teach.

## MEDICAL MASTERWORK, *NURSING THE INSANE* (1908)

Superintendent Selden Talcott held a vision for the Middletown Hospital and oversaw every facet of the asylum's operation, but Clara Barrus stood equal to Talcott as visionary and a punctilious apostle of standards. She was also charged with inspiring the hospital's army of nurses and converting a compassionate and holistic mission into specific, caregiving directives.

Barrus was neither a nurse nor a male doctor; *Nursing the Insane*'s author was listed as Clara Barrus, M.D., Woman Assistant Physician in the Middletown State Homeopathic Hospital, Middletown, N.Y. Composed in an elegant style, her book may be the most comprehensive, enlightened, and holistic nursing manual ever written.

The modern era opts for the quick and superficial fix. Rather than engaging with those overwhelmed by trauma and anguish, today's mental health caregivers medicalize their patients' plights. Demand for convenience and pharmaceutical profit nullifies the spiritual struggles of the mentally ill. We know that abhorrent and inexplicable behaviors are merely expressive of traumatic impact and that when these are suppressed with narcotics, anxiolytic, and neuroleptic drugs, all possibility of progress halts. Yet Clara Barrus's ethic, a warrior-like commitment to empowering rather than obstructing her patients in solving problems of living, is now all but obsolete. Her masterwork could not be written today.

We recall Thomas Szasz's insistence that "our adversaries are not demons, witches, fate, or mental illness. We have no enemy whom we can fight, exorcise, or dispel by 'cure.' What we do have are problems in living."

*Nursing the Insane* reveals that Barrus's arsenal of weapons included not drugs but determination; compassion; moral authority; psychological, nutritional, medical, and pragmatic advice; and wisdom. *Nursing the Insane* is also a window into the workaday duties and onerous challenges facing a hospital's preeminent workforce—its nurses.

Though the word *medicine* is used, its denotation as homeopathy does not appear in the book. This bespeaks Barrus's laser-like focus on the nursing function, which did not include prescribing. Her aim was to instill among nurses not only respect for physicians in their elevated role as prescribers but also psychological astuteness in their own dealings with patients. The following excerpts from Barrus's four-hundred-page text are chosen to evoke the warmth of her personality and the breadth of her perspective.

## The Ideal Nurse

*[The ideal nurse] is one whose bodily presence breathes health and cleanliness, one of quiet garb, of noiseless step, of soothing hand, of cheerful spirit, and of hopeful heart, and one of ready but judicious sympathy. We must not forget the "low and gentle voice," which, if it be "an excellent thing in woman," is especially so in a nurse. To these qualities must be added punctuality, truthfulness, patience, obedience, caution, courage, a spirit of untiring helpfulness, a vigilance that never sleeps, a sympathy that is inexhaustible, and a tact that can cope successfully with the most trying and complex of situations.*

*The nurse for mental and nervous invalids needs to be especially careful to conceal prejudices, to beware of showing favoritism, to conquer resentment* and antipathies, to study the art of peacemaking, to learn when to speak and when to refrain from speaking, when to act and when not to act. She must learn humility and forbearance; in short, she must so cultivate the virtues that she becomes but little lower than the angels. And here I am reminded of what George Eliot says: "To be anxious about a soul that is always snapping at you must be left to the saints of the earth," and you are no saints, but just mortal men and women who have undertaken a work that makes continual demands upon your moral as well as your physical strength. I would not have you think I underestimate these demands. I would only try to help you cope with them as I believe you wish to do, worthily and well.

## The Progressive Nurse

The progressive nurse is always on the alert to learn how she can grow more and more efficient, and here I wish to caution the experienced nurse against thinking there is nothing else for her to learn, no newer and better methods to adopt, no truer application of the old methods. Those of us who have been in the work many years have to acknowledge that some patients get well in spite of, rather than because of, our efforts; and that others drift into chronicity because we are wanting in the energy and resourcefulness to rouse them to activity and to mental restoration. Have we not seen patients that have been regarded as hopeless unaccountably take a favorable turn and surprise every one by getting well . . . some subtle influences have been at work of which we are not aware. These experiences make us see the necessity of studying into and revising methods needing revision. . . . We need to keep step with the advance bring made in the study and treatment of nervous and mental disorders. Antiquated ideas and methods must be cast aside for newer, more enlightened views and methods; routine must give place to individualization. The necessary red tape of an institution must be supplemented by variety and freshness. We must get out of ruts, look at our patients with a fresh eye, and bestir ourselves to try something different if old ways have proved ineffectual.

## Against Discouragement

We have a right to console ourselves when we see, in spite of the utmost care, that a patient has drifted into the condition of chronicity. But be sure that *the patient has received your utmost care, your best efforts, your unfailing efforts, to stimulate and to restore. Even then, be careful how you regard a given case as incurable. Better err on the side of hoping against hope than to relax in any particular efforts toward bringing about a recovery. Keep alive your own optimism even in the face of discouragement. Optimism is infectious.*

*One sometimes hears a nurse say: "It is so discouraging caring for these chronic cases. If we could only have something worth working for!" Let me again and again warn you against regarding a patient as incurable; but even granted that a given case is hopeless, or suppose your entire service is composed of seemingly hopeless cases, what then? In the first place it is your duty to minister to a chronic patient's physical wants just as conscientiously as though she were the most promising of patients. The bodily functions should be regularly and closely watched, and any irregularities promptly reported to the physician. Do not take it upon yourself to decide as to their importance; let the physician do that. Your duty is to observe and report. The patient's appetite, the sleep, the functions of urination and of defecation, the menstrual function, the condition of the skin, the habits, tendencies, false beliefs, conduct—all these, and many others not enumerated, should be intelligently and regularly scrutinized by you, and any departure from the normal promptly announced to the attending physician.*

*I have seen a new and energetic nurse take charge of a room full of chronic patients who had been allowed by a former nurse to eat with their fingers, shoving in the food in a most repulsive way; in a few weeks' time I have seen that nurse's painstaking efforts rewarded by an orderly set of patients decorously feeding themselves with spoons from neatly arranged trays, the same cases that other nurses had declared could not be made to do differently. But this transformation was not effected without patience, perseverance, tact, and a careful study of, and attention to, each individual patient; for what works well with one will often have no effect upon another.*

## Rules to Observe When on Duty

*In every way that lies in our power we should seek to individualize each patient; keep him alive to his own personality; do not class him as one of a mass; he has his individual life to live, his own hopes, fears, and desires; his* own place in creation; and it is our duty at all times to respect this, to help him to appreciate it, if, by reason of his disordered intellect, he is in danger of forgetting it. Always call patients by name, do not speak of them as "he," or "she"; let each feel that he is somebody, a particular somebody—not a mere something grouped in a mass and called "the patients."

Right here, in your own field, are the battles you are called upon to fight with disease and delusion. The enemy's ranks are all around you; one must contend with indifference and sloth; with depression and stupefaction; with long-standing habits; with perverseness, malice, error, blindness; with uncleanliness of deed, word, and thought. You are, in fact, encompassed by a large army of evil passions uncontrolled, with all their uncertain and dangerous tendencies, but you are enlisted against them, and so long as you stay in the service, it is your duty to rally your forces and to rout the offenders.

## Hygiene of Wards and Infirmaries
In ventilating one needs to guard against the fallacy that cold air is necessarily pure air, and that warm air is necessarily impure. The temperature has nothing to do with the purity or the impurity of the air. A room which has not been heated or ventilated for weeks may be filled with cold, stale air unfit to breathe. A ward does not need to be cold and uncomfortable in order to be sanitary. By changing the air frequently and closing up between times, the halls can be kept hygienic as well as comfortable. Fireplaces are the best means of ventilation, but there are few of them in many hospitals, and these few are seldom in use. But even when not in use, if kept open, they furnish an exit for the impure air. A fire in the grate, by causing a constant draught of air to ascend the chimney, and a constant quantity of fresh air to descend as well, is one of the most effective means of ventilation.

## Observation of Symptoms
It is the nurse's duty to report all subjective complaints whether she believes them to be real, exaggerated, minimized, or feigned; but if she has good ground for believing them to be simulated, it is proper for her to mention such grounds. Let it be remembered that these very subjective complaints, even when exaggerated or feigned, may be of the utmost importance to the

*physician. In early cases of mental alienation it is especially important to note the complaints of changes in the organic sensations, for these are often of such a nature as to interfere with the combination of sensations that make up the patient's individuality, and the study of these is often of the greatest help in tracing the beginnings of the alteration of the ego; in other words, of seeing the bridge across which the person passes from sanity to insanity.*

*General appearance of patient:*

> *Dress—tidy, untidy, clean, unclean, precise, slovenly, fantastic, fastened imperfectly or carelessly regarding decency; droppings of food; shoes, where most worn, if disorders in gait are noted.*
>
> *Behavior—timid, reckless, modest, bold, docile, unruly, mild, boisterous, meek, boastful, indifferent to surroundings, interested, overcurious, mischievous, restless, apathetic, occupied, idle, destructive, oversensitive, peaceable, threatening, flighty, poor control.*
>
> *State of nutrition and apparent or real weight and height—emaciated, slender, well nourished, stout, obese, dwarfish, short, medium, tall, very tall.*
>
> *Complexion—fair, dark, medium, sallow, ruddy, florid.*
>
> *Hair—color, texture, quantity, baldness (general or local).*
>
> *Eyes—color, expression, appearance of pupils.*
>
> *Facial expression—calm, happy, anxious, worried, suffering, dejected, elated, egotistical, shrinking, pinched, tranquil, dull, stupid, bewildered, besotted, delirious, dazed, convulsed, etc.*
>
> *Carriage and posture of body—walking erect, bent, staggering; sitting erect, stooping; lounging, lolling about, etc.; lying down, apathetic, restless, sliding down in bed, etc. Manner of moving about, impairment of motion, etc.*

*Objective signs in special organs and parts: Note if there is anything unusual in appearance or condition of head and face, and organs of special sense; neck or throat; chest; back or abdomen; extremities; genital organs; skin.*

*Subjective complaints: Pain, tenderness, abnormal sensations, numbness, nausea, vertigo, etc. Is pain sharp, dull, burning, stinging, darting, band-like, needle-like, constant, intermittent, spasmodic?*

*Mental state—intellectual field: Conscious, unconscious, dull, alert, rational, irrational, delusions, hallucinations, illusions, hobbies, queer ways, perversions, lapses in memory, fabrications, disorders in speech, misapprehending of persons and surroundings, suicidal or homicidal tendencies, self-accusations, ideas of reference, or of undue or unfair influence.*

*Emotional field: Self-controlled, or rapidly changing and uncontrolled emotions; happy, sad, cheerful, joyous, morose, irascible; signs of affection, love, rage, fear, dread, hopefulness, jealousy, envy, sympathy, merriment, grief, zeal, ennui; feeling of unreality, credulity, doubt, aspiration, elation, depression, hesitation, indecision, timidity, anxiety, irritation, contentment, pride, humility, admiration, patience, scorn, rebellion, abhorrence, contempt, disgust, pity, impatience, expansion and ease, or contraction and tension; sensitive to the beautiful, the sublime, the comic, etc.*

## Care of Special Medical Cases

Apart from their mental condition, asylum patients could also, of course, be inflicted with all sorts of other disorders and sometimes fell grievously ill with challenging conditions. Doctors and nurses needed to be prepared for many diseases in their acute and chronic manifestations, including:

*Cerebrospinal meningitis—The treatment of cerebro-spinal meningitis should aim to secure good nutrition, free bowels, thorough ventilation, darkness, and quiet. Noise, light, and even the lightest touch are likely to increase the spasms. Ice bags to the head and spine help to relieve the pain. Although the disease is not very communicable, the patient should be isolated.*

*Influenza (la grippe)—In the treatment of influenza isolation is advisable. At the beginning a hot bath and hot lemonade are given to induce sweating, and such remedies as are prescribed by the physician.*

*Tuberculosis—The care of the tubercular patient may be summed up in a few words—the prevention of the spread of the disease, supplying an abundance of fresh air continuously, teaching the patient to breathe properly, furnishing sufficient quantities of nourishing and easily digested food, suitable clothing, bathing him frequently, and in securing moderate exercise in some cases and complete rest for others, and very little if any internal medication.*

*The nurse for the tubercular insane has to contend with extra difficulties, for in many cases she can get no cooperation on the part of the patient. Some patients will swallow their sputum and others will expectorate wherever they wish—on the floor, bedding, behind radiators, in their handkerchiefs, or on their petticoats, in the faces of the attendants and of other patients, and so on. Some will rub the expectorated matter in their hair or beards.*

## Amusement of Patients

*Did you ever hear of a "Giggle class"? Even this, as silly as it seems, may be made beneficial, and it certainly is amusing.*

*Ten persons are asked to stand in a circle. Beginning at one point, one says "Ha!" the next follows, and so on around. The next time around, "Ha, Ha!" more rapidly, and again more Ha's and still more rapidly, until all lose their turn in their effort to catch it up, and so, what started out to be a mechanical giggle becomes a downright laugh in good earnest all round.*

*Some of these suggestions may seem very trivial, but at the risk of their appearing so, I mention them with the hope that, even if the ones suggested are not tried, they will at least put you in mind of others that may appeal to you as better and more suited to the particular cases with which you have to deal.*

Well in advance of Thomas Szasz, Clara Barrus stood against the notion that insanity is readily assessed. In *Nursing the Insane* she continues:

## There Is No Standard of Sanity and Insanity

*Certain beliefs and manifestations that would be madness if held by a person who has received a liberal education are simply the natural result of ignorance and credulity, or of false theology, or of low associations, in another. Each person has to be judged according to his race, class, family, educational, religious, and social standing. Many sane persons have delusions; that is, they hold false beliefs; but these are the result of insufficient teaching and training, and so we call them sane delusions. In the days of the Salem witchcraft the belief in witches was held by a large number of sane persons, and even today in certain rural districts of New York State there are whole communities where the people still believe in witches.*

*Erroneous as are their views, we know they are not insane, they are merely ignorant. But if a person who has been liberally educated, who has had the advantages of travel and of intercourse with the best minds, through personal relations and through books, comes to express the belief that she is bewitched, that the doctors are casting a spell upon her, and that all sorts of tortures are being inflicted by unseen agencies, we can readily see that she is suffering from an insane delusion. It is contrary to what she believed when her mind worked in a healthy way, and she has lost the power to recognize the fallacy of such an opinion.*

*Mental disorders assume a variety of forms, according to the character and extent of disturbance of the different mental functions; the trouble may be chiefly in disturbances in perception, giving rise to hallucinations and illusions, or in the intellectual sphere, giving rise to disturbances of memory, disturbances in the formation of ideas, of the train of thought, of the reasoning and judgment, of the rapidity of thought, or of the consciousness; or the difficulty may be in the emotional sphere; or it may be in disturbances of volition and action.*

*The human being is a very complex creature, made up of a complicated body in which all the organs and parts working together comprise the individual life. We cannot, as I have said, think of the body and mind as separate; they act and react upon each other too intimately to consider them apart except for convenience in speaking. When body and mind work in harmony, when the functions are properly performed, when the impressions that come to us from without, and the sensations that arise within, are correctly interpreted, that is health—health of body and health of mind. Of course there are variations within the limits of health; no one is perfectly sound in every part at all times, but we are governed by the predominating conditions in speaking of health or disease. When, however, there is a prolonged departure from the normal and harmonious workings of the various parts, disease exists, and we name the disease in accordance with whatever part bears the brunt of the disturbance, whether it be heart, lungs, stomach, intestines, muscles, blood vessels, nerves, or brain. Yet, let me repeat, we need to keep in mind that none of these parts works independently, and all are to varying degrees affected by disturbances in one another.*

## LIFE AFTER MIDDLETOWN

Clara Barrus left Middletown Hospital after seventeen years and in 1912 opened a private sanatorium in Pelham, New York, where she served until her retirement in 1914. In her later years she became a psychoanalyst, naturalist, and devotee of the conservationist John Burroughs.

An imbalance I hope to redress concerns how much better-known Barrus is as the muse of a naturalist than as a homeopathic physician and psychiatrist. Yet it cannot be denied that John Burroughs was famous in his day and a transcendent figure in her life.

Barrus met John Burroughs while she was practicing medicine and became associated with him for almost two decades, until his death in 1921. She was Burroughs's friend, secretary, biographer, and almost constant traveling companion. When he died Barrus was named his literary executor. Among other works, she edited two posthumous volumes of Burroughs's essays and wrote *Whitman and Burroughs, Comrades* about the relationship between Burroughs and poet Walt Whitman.

Following a long illness, Clara Barrus died on April 4, 1931.

# 10

## Disciples and Satellites of the Mother Church

*And when I am forgotten, as I shall be, and asleep in dull*
*cold marble, where no mention of me more must be heard*
*of, say I taught thee.*
WILLIAM SHAKESPEARE, *HENRY VIII*,
ACT III, SCENE 2

Beyond his many gifts, Seldon Talcott was a respected mentor whose disciples tended to emulate his career pathway via serving a stint at Ward's Island before working with him at Middletown. They would then cycle through either Westborough Insane Hospital in Massachusetts, or New York's Fergus Falls State Hospital, or Gowanda Homeopathic State Hospital before opening a sanatorium of their own. Talcott's methods influenced care of the mentally ill from the late 1800s through the beginning of the twentieth century, and the following is a sampling of his importance.

### N. EMMONS PAINE

N. Emmons Paine, an assistant physician at Middletown, was one of Selden Talcott's most prominent disciples and promoted homeopathy's position within the Association of Medical Superintendents of American Institutions for the Insane. He was recruited to be the first superintendent of a successful asylum—Westborough Insane Hospital, regarded as the second homeopathic hospital in the nation—in 1886. Westborough's opening census of 204 patients constituted an over-flow from crowded hospitals in the neighboring towns of Taunton, Northampton, Danvers, and Worcester.

Emmons was a long-standing, progressive member of the American Psychiatric Association and committed to elevating the psychiatric edu-cation of asylum doctors. When he was appointed as lecturer in insan-ity at Boston University Medical School in 1888, he followed the lead of Talcott, who directed New York Homeopathic Medical College students through rotations at Middletown, by offering the same kind of educational experience at Westborough for his Boston University medical students.

Paine was handy with instruments, and, as Talcott noted, in 1879 he introduced an improvement to the Nelaton rubber catheter that rendered the nasogastric tube less likely to cause aspiration. The widely used device came to be called Paine's naso-stomach feeding tube.[1]

In 1892, Dr. Paine opened a private sanatorium in his home, the Newton Nervine Asylum. Though it began modestly with four patients, over the next ten years three buildings were added to accommodate a total of twenty-one patients.[2]

## WESTBOROUGH STATE HOMEOPATHIC HOSPITAL

Much like Middletown Hospital, Westborough Hospital relied chiefly on homeopathy, diet, hydrotherapy, and rest in the treatment of patients. As shown in the hospital's annual reports compared to the other state hospitals, Westborough recorded a high recovery rate into the turn of the century.[3]

A nursing school was established at Westborough in 1891, and the first female doctor at the hospital was appointed as assistant physician in 1893. Several buildings were added during this period, including a mortuary, staff housing, and Talbot House, a striking Colonial Revival

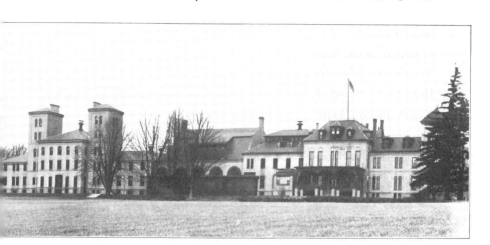

**Westborough State Homeopathic Hospital Grand View.
Number of beds, 1,235; number of patients treated during
prior fiscal year, 1,855. There are more than sixty buildings
grouped about the extensive grounds.**
Courtesy of the American Institute of Homeopathy Council on Medical Education,
from *Hospitals and Sanatoriums of the Homoeopathic School of Medicine* (1916)

building designed by Rand, Taylor, Kendall, and Stevens. (Rand also
designed the iconic Kirkbride building at Worcester.)

In 1903 two satellite colonies for quiet chronic patients were established on the south shore of Lake Chauncey, the Warren Farm Colony
for men (1903) and the Richmond Colony for women. Wards for
chronic disturbed patients and a large kitchen building were added to
the main complex in 1906. The property eventually expanded to more
than 650 acres, much of it farmed to stock the hospital's food supply
until the program was ended in the 1970s. The institution was renamed
Westborough State Hospital in 1907.[4]

As in so many hospitals, over time a move to new programs aimed
at research, general health, prevention, and outpatient services reduced
the time allotted for individual care. The role allotted to homeopathy
declined, especially with expansion of the hospital's census. When the
Governor and Council's Committee visited Westborough in 1945, the
patient population had swelled to 1,730, well beyond the normal capacity of 1,332.

Due to the effects of World War II, staffing levels also fell, reaching a low of 239, with 210 vacancies. Many buildings were seriously over-crowded, and several, including the old 1848 Lyman School, were noted as firetraps. Tragically, admission of a few, poorly supervised, criminally insane women resulted in the murder of a number of other patients. The hospital was closed in 2010 in anticipation of a new Worcester State Hospital opening in 2012. Almost all of the buildings at Westborough State Hospital were demolished in 2019.[5]

## BUTLER ASYLUM

The forerunner to today's Butler Hospital was the Butler Asylum, a Providence, Rhode Island, facility that gained renown and gener-ous funding under the twenty-two-year reign (1845–1867) of its first superintendent, Dr. Isaac Ray. A former Harvard Medical School student and Medical School of Maine at Bowdoin College graduate, Dr. Ray was one of the original founders of what is now the American Psychiatric Association (APA) and a pioneer in the fields of medi-cal jurisprudence and forensic psychology. In Selden Talcott fashion Dr. Ray toured and investigated the asylums of Europe prior to super-vising Butler Asylum.

The same question we asked in relation to Richard Patterson's asy-lum at Bellevue Place may now be asked about Butler: How is it that an essentially hand-holding, moral care–espousing asylum could acquire so stellar a reputation for doing the impossible—healing the mentally ill? Hydrotherapy, recreation, bucolic surroundings, and attentiveness would not account for it. The case may be circumstantial in regard to Richard Patterson, but in regard to Butler there is no mistake—the hos-pital's secret weapon was homeopathy.

Butler was founded in 1844 as Rhode Island's first exclusively men-tal health hospital. Industrialist Cyrus Butler donated heavily to the hospital, wherefore it was named in his honor. Businessman philanthro-pist Nicholas Brown Jr. also bequeathed a substantial sum to construct a mental asylum, money that was used to fund the early hospital. Butler Hospital's 1844 Gothic Revival complex was listed on the National Register of Historic Places in 1976.

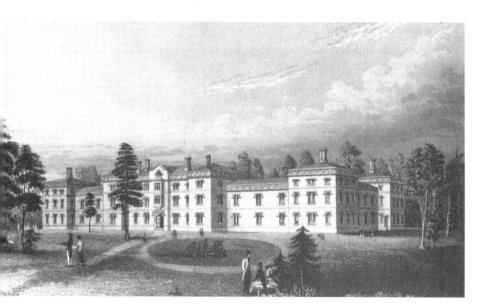

1886 engraving of Butler Asylum

The hospital boasted a tennis court, putting green, horseshoe field, athletic field, baseball field, and library, along with facilities for basket making, hooked rug work, carpentry, and use of a power jigsaw. Patient creations were sold to subsidize purchase of supplies and equipment.

In 1926 the Trustees and Superintendent of Butler Hospital published a text, *The Butler Hospital: Its Story,* within which a visit by Dorothea Dix is recorded.

First, she struck upon scenes of misery almost beyond belief, scenes in deep stone dungeons without light or air, where insane persons were entombed in living death. Second, she found that "there existed in the City of Providence a small asylum, conducted on wise and humane principles, but totally inadequate to the demands made upon it." Miss Dix resolved that an appeal to the wealthy and humane for the immediate enlargement of this asylum was a step that must be taken.[6]

*The Butler Hospital: Its Story* expresses pride in the hospital's nutrition, stating, "The most scrupulous attention is given to dietetics.

Wholesome, health-giving food was prepared by experienced cooks under the direction of trained dietitians."[7]

At Butler Hospital the patient was left as free as possible, though carefully watched by nurses when necessary. The object was to retain him or her in their ward by persuasion, if possible, not by mechanical barriers.

Its wide-ranging treatments, unrestrained by dogma or cost, included hydrotherapy, hours of relaxation in warm water, ice packs on the head, hot drinks, a quartz lamp to treat skin lesions and other disorders, surgical operations, and "treatments of every kind" as needed "with no thought whatever of expense. Speedy recovery is the only consideration."[8] The hospital also pioneered a committed outpatient aftercare program for discharged patients.

Following is further description from *The Butler Hospital: Its Story.*

*Broad lawns, shaded by century-old trees, surround all the buildings, and give the patients a stimulating outlook. . . .*

*Everything is done to help patients quiet their unstrung nerves, to make them feel at home and at rest.*

*And the result? You will see it as you pass from the wards where newly arrived, acutely ill patients are, to the other wards where, more and more, the patients are regaining their rationality, finding again the true relations of things, tasting life once more.*

*The first step in treating the mentally ill is, of course, learning the history of the patient, studying his present condition, and making a thorough diagnosis and prognosis of the case. When a patient enters, no matter what his apparent condition, he goes to bed for at least three days, during which time he is under constant observation. The attending psychiatrist, in making his study of the case, takes every step to make the patient realize that he is in a hospital, and that the object of his coming is to effect a cure.*

*Before the final decision as to treatment is made, the case is summarized before the staff, of which the superintendent is head. The patient is brought before the staff. Later the attending physician goes over his recommendations with the staff. After this thorough consultation, the treatment of the case is begun.*[9]

Concerning effective treatment modalities among which the attending psychiatrist and his staff could choose, *Its Story* is silent. But here is a clue: For more than two years (January 14, 1867, until June 30, 1869) there happened to be on staff a physician who was one of the world's foremost psychiatric homeopaths, an ardent disciple of Selden Talcott and the author of a renowned homeopathic text, *Insanity and Its Treatment: Lectures on the Treatment of Insanity and Kindred Nervous Diseases.* This was Samuel Worcester. A connection exists between APA founder Isaac Ray, who attended Harvard Medical College, and Samuel Worcester, who graduated from there. Harvard Medical College's connection to homeopathy can be said to go back to its origins. In 1783 the college's founding faculty consisted of three members, one of whom, Benjamin Waterhouse, was professor of physic (as medicine was then known), serving in that capacity until 1812. The era's zeitgeist produced Samuel Hahnemann and his theory of homeopathy; and the English physician Edward Jenner (1749–1823), who had begun experimenting with small doses of a "like to cure like" cowpox disease to prevent smallpox infection. Demonstrating conclusively that homeopathic inoculation provided protection against the disease, Waterhouse, an early adopter of Edward Jenner's original (non-antibiotic carrying) cowpox vaccine, successfully vaccinated his children with it.

Though beyond the scope of *Sane Asylums,* Harvard's connection to homeopathy merits a mention. Harvard is not in name a homeopathic school, but medical instruction there prior to the Flexner Report was so infused with the values of transcendentalism and the influence of Emanuel Swedenborg that it can be presumed to have included homeopathy.* The beloved physician of Louisa May Alcott, for example,

---

*The 1910 Flexner Report, sponsored by the Carnegie Foundation, is generally taught as having been educationally beneficial, having demanded that medical schools adhere to rigorous standards. In an alternative narrative the report is notorious for having warped medical education. In its wake, long-espoused, patient-centered standards were discarded so that profit-first (spun as "scientific") directives could take their place. Rockefeller's minions infiltrated and commandeered medical school boards. Abetted by a well-funded advertising campaign, his toxic oil-refining by-product pharmaceuticals flooded the marketplace. What had been customary reliance on effective and side effect free homeopathic and botanical medicine grew passé. Numerous medical schools, homeopathic schools among them, were forced to close.

a homeopath by the name of Conrad Wesselhoeft, was a 1911 graduate of Harvard Medical School.[10]

## SAMUEL WORCESTER

Best known for a classic homeopathic work on the treatment of mental illness and nervous disease, Samuel Worcester, M.D., was a descendant of doctors and ministers. His father, Samuel H. Worcester, M.D., of Salem, Massachusetts, suffered for months in his youth from a scrofulous affection of the eyes. Finding him "permanently unfit" for further study, his physician, Dr. John C. Warren of Boston, referred him to Dr. Hans Burch Gram of New York, the Danish homeopath who had brought Hahnemann's system to New England. Gram soon cured the senior Worcester, thus enabling him to enter college.[11]

The younger Samuel Worcester matriculated at Harvard Medical College, graduating in 1868. Prior to that, in 1865 he was appointed Medical Cadet United States Army and ordered on duty to the National General Hospital in Baltimore. There he remained until the conclusion of the Civil War, when due to military service–related ill health he was honorably discharged.

Soon upon leaving Baltimore, Worcester was appointed assistant physician to the Butler Hospital for the Insane in Providence, Rhode Island, in January 1867, remaining there as we have learned until June 1869. During the remainder of the summer Worcester practiced at Massachusetts Eye and Ear Infirmary in Boston, after which he secured a teaching position at the medical college in Philadelphia. In April 1870, Worcester entered general practice in Concord, Massachusetts, later relocating to Burlington, Vermont, and establishing a private practice.

In the winter of 1879 to 1880, Worcester prepared and delivered a series of lectures for the senior class of the Boston University School of Medicine. These were revised and again delivered at the session of 1880 to 1881. Responding to entreaties from the students for a comprehensive work on insanity, Worcester made additions and further revisions to the lectures. With a dedication to Selden Talcott these were published as *Insanity and Its Treatment: Lectures on the*

*Treatment of Insanity and Kindred Nervous Diseases* in 1882. According to Jonathan Davidson's compilation,[12] Worcester had a hand in the establishment of the Westborough Asylum, being one of the first to propose its creation. Together with Selden Talcott he testified at the Garfield assassination trial. Despite speaking for the defense, like Talcott he found the defendant Charles Guiteau not to be insane.

A contributor to various medical journals, Worcester was also associate editor of the *New England Medical Gazette,* Department of Psychological Medicine. Worcester was active in the Massachusetts Homeopathic Medical Society, the Vermont Homeopathic Medical Society, the American Institute of Homeopathy, and an honorary member of the Homeopathic Medical Society of the State of New York.

Worcester's *Insanity and Its Treatment* stands out for its clarity, the range of its references (Worcester's claim of having consulted several hundred volumes of source material is borne out by the text), and the practicality of his teachings in support of Hahnemann, that remedy choice could vary within a single diagnosis.

To provide a sense of Worcester's teaching the following section from *Insanity* concerning melancholia and mania has been chosen.

*For my notes upon the medical treatment of this as well as the other forms of insanity I am largely indebted to the kindness of Dr. Selden H. Talcott, Superintendent of the State Homoeopathic Hospital for the Insane at Middletown, New York, who has furnished me with some of the results obtained at that institution.*

*Melancholia and mania, alternating as they do so frequently in some patients, often require similar remedies. It is not the name of a disease nor, indeed, the supposed pathological condition, which must always be a matter of uncertainty, but the array and totality of the symptoms that indicates the choice of a drug. Still for purposes of convenience we sometimes group under the name of a disease, certain drugs most often of service in the cure of that disease.*

*Digitalis rises to prominence in this connection, not so much by reason of the fame it has acquired in "the books," but on account of the effects following its use when homoeopathically indicated. It is mostly of use when the patient is in a dull lethargic condition; the pupils are dilated to their widest, yet all sensibility to light or to touch seems lost; the pulse is full, regular, or but slightly intermittent and* very slow. *The slow pulse is the grand characteristic, and upon this indication Digitalis may be given with much assurance that relief will follow speedily, if relief be possible. We notice that the Digitalis patient, when rallying from his melancholic stupor, often moans a good deal, and his eyes are all afloat in tears. Relief, however, speedily follows the bursting of the lachrymal fountains.*

*It has long been supposed and advocated that Aurum metallicum was the princely remedy for suicidal melancholia. But the experience at Middletown does not fully sustain this idea. Dr. Talcott says: "Aurum has often been prescribed in such cases, but usually without good results. Another remedy which we have tried repeatedly has generally hit the case most happily, and that remedy is Arsenicum. My mind has been exercised in solving the mystery of Arsenicum's happy effect in cases of suicidal tendency, while the much-vaunted Aurum has repeatedly failed. Our conclusion is this: the patients whom Arsenicum has relieved have been those whose physical condition would warrant the administration of that drug. They have been much emaciated with wretched appetites; a dry, red tongue; shriveled skin; haggard and anxious in appearance, and evidently great bodily suffering. It would seem as if the mental unrest of these patients was due, in the main, to physical disease, and consequent exhaustion, and their desire to commit suicide is evidently for the purpose of putting an end to their temporal distresses. On the other hand the suicidal patients whom Aurum has seemed to benefit are usually in fair health, physically; but have experienced some unfortunate disaster of the affections, or have had trouble with friends; they fancy they have been slighted, persecuted and wronged, and out of revenge or disgust for the irksome trials of life seek an untimely end by their own hands.*[13]

Here is Worcester discussing hysteria:

*In our treatment we should distinguish between the hysterical condition and the hysterical fit. The latter is by far the more easily controlled as you would suppose.*

---

*Note: in my own practice suicidal patients of the physically robust type as Talcott describes have done wonderfully well with Aurum met.

*Asa foetida* will help in hysteria of young women complaining of a gone-empty feeling in the epigastrium, which is not a pain, but "it hurts them." Pulsations in the same place, which come on about eleven o'clock and make them feel faint.

For the nervous condition:

General increased sensibility: *Ignatia amara, Cypripedium pubescens, Sepia* and *Stramonium*

Heightened sensitiveness: *Cocculus indicus, Stramoniumim, Platina, Pulsatilla nigricans, Aconitum napellus,* and *Nux vomica*

Irritability and impatience: *Gelsemium sempervirens, Sepia, Pulsatilla nigricans, Nux vomica., Hyoscyamus niger*

Variable disposition: *Ignatia amara, Pulsatalla nigricans, Stramonium, Moschus, Platina, Sepia*

Constant brooding: *Nux vomica, Ignatia amara, Sepia*

Constant and excessive dread: *Aconitum napellus, Pulsatilla nigricans, Platina*

Fidgety expectation: *Valeriana officinalis*

Persistent silence, or constant moaning and lamentation: *Nux vomica*

Bodily Conditions and Symptoms

Constant troublesome sinking at the stomach: *Asa foetida, Cimicifuga racemosa, Gelsemium sempervirens, Hydrastis canadensis, Ignatia amara*

Shortness of breath and cold feet: *Calcarea carbonica*

Oppression of chest: *Moschus* and *Ignatia amara*

Sleeplessness: *Cypripedium pubescens, Gelsem., Ignat., Nux vomica*

If we consider the cause so far as ascertainable, we find fright: *Aconitum napellus;* disappointment and grief: *Ignatia amara;* prolonged watching and nursing: *Nux vomica, Ignatia amara, Cypripedium pubescens;* intense or continual mental strain: *Cypripedium pubescens, Phosphorus, China officinalis, Nux vomica;* ovarian or uterine irritation: *Caulophyllum thalictroides, Cimicifuga racemosa, Belladonna*

*Belladonna* will often be of marked benefit in controlling the convulsive paroxysm.

*I can of course touch only briefly on the indications for the proper remedy, for as hysteria may simulate any disease under the sun, you will find that no disease will require a more searching study of your Materia Medica, but above everything it is necessary that your patients should be built up by plenty of good nourishing food to which they often object; and should be placed in as pleasant a situation as possible, free from care, anxiety and worry.*[14]

## GOWANDA HOMEOPATHIC STATE HOSPITAL

In the 1890s in the western part of New York state demand had arisen for accommodations and homeopathic care for the mentally ill. While large numbers of such persons were annually committed to state hospitals, provision was made for such special care and treatment was scant. Swinging into action the Committee on Medical Legislation of the State Homeopathic Medical Society achieved enactment of chapter 707, Laws of 1894, signed by the governor on May 15 of that year. By provisions of the statute, a 500-acre tract known as Collins Farm was set apart in the Erie County town of Collins so that a second state homeopathic hospital for the insane could be established. During 1897 the first buildings listed were completed and equipped (see photo on facing page).

In May 1897, Dr. George Allen was appointed the first superintendent of Gowanda Hospital. After his health failed and he died in November of the same year, the Board of Managers tapped the expertise and cachet of Middletown Hospital by appointing Dr. Daniel H. Arthur, formerly assistant physician at Middletown, as superintendent. Dr. Arthur, in turn, appointed Dr. George Francis Adams of Westborough, an 1888 graduate of Hahnemann Medical College of Chicago, as first assistant physician.

Of Dr. Adams we know the following: His career began with seven years in practice in Pulaski, New York, before he became chief of staff of the state hospital at Westborough for three years. He then became connected with Gowanda Homeopathic State Hospital, contributing his services there for six years. His expertise lay in the diagnosis and treatment of melancholia and depression.

The hospital in Gowanda became operative August 9, 1898, on which date forty-seven patients were received. Soon an additional seven patients

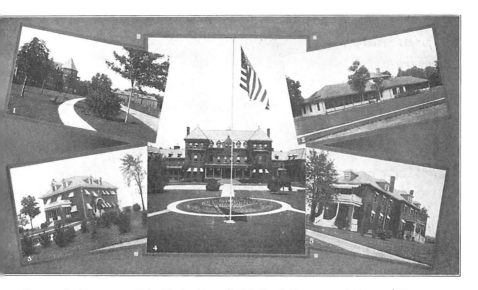

Gowanda Homeopathic State Hospital 1. East Group and Nurses' Home
2. Pavilion for Aged Women 3. Superintendent's Residence
4. Administration Building 5. Staff House
Courtesy of the American Institute of Homeopathy, from *Hospitals and
Sanatoriums of the Homoeopathic School of Medicine* (1916)

were added. In 1898 the managers reported: "The board feels gratified
in its accomplishment. It has labored long and zealously to secure to the
homeopathic school of medicine and to the adherents of homeopathy a
hospital in which they or their friends, if afflicted with this calamitous disease of insanity, could be treated according to their teachings and belief."

Additional buildings constructed during 1898 were a powerhouse,
water tower, water supply pipes, and a hospital wing known as the West
Group, confusingly referred to at times as the West Wing. Predating its
construction was a separate wing of the hospital adjacent to the nurses'
wing that may (perhaps humorously) have come to be referred to as the
East Group following the addition of the West Group.

Gowanda Homeopathic State Hospital West Group was described
in the 1930s as having 1,254 beds, with 1,429 patients that year treated
by six house staff, and 4.1 percent deaths. Staffing even then included
ten homeopathic physicians from the western New York area working
as consultants (which is why the medical complex was called the West

Group); they continued to treat patients under strict homeopathic auspices.

The medical complex consisted of two-story wings projecting from the main building, two three-story pavilion-style buildings, two pavilions for patients with tuberculosis (TB), powerhouse, laundry, kitchen, main dining room building, smaller dining rooms in several buildings, farm, workshops, nurses' home, storeroom, amusement hall/auditorium, main staff house, and superintendent's residence, all built prior to 1946.

Gowanda also had a hospital nursing school that trained employees for the facility. A graduate program was held every year on the hospital grounds in September. Nurses wore the traditional nurses' white cap and a seersucker dress with a white apron. The average class was coed. Many of the orderlies at Gowanda were Seneca Indians who lived on the Cattaraugus Indian Reservation property that abutted the state hospital property. The hospital maintained an archery range, a three-hole golf course, a pond stocked with fish, and a recreation center with two showings of movies on Saturdays.

Admissions to the hospital usually occurred during the day, and usually by court order. They were isolated from other patients for thirty days for observation and testing. Mentally ill patients were frequently disoriented by previous experiences, and thirty days of a more peaceful environment generally improved their demeanor or revealed problems. Patients were disoriented for various reasons ranging from mental disease or experiences of war to loss of family, homelessness, job loss, and other traumatic life events. Patients judged to be criminally insane were not retained at Gowanda but instead sent to Matteawan State Hospital for the criminally insane or Dannemora State Hospital for Insane Convicts.[15]

## CINCINNATI SANITARIUM

From 1880 to 1903, Dr. Orpheus Everts was superintendent of a private sane asylum, the Cincinnati Sanitarium, which three physicians (likely homeopaths) had established in 1873. As we have seen with other such asylums, designating it specifically as a homeopathic facility was not always appropriate.

Located in the city's College Hill neighborhood, Cincinnati Sanitarium was the first private psychiatric facility in the United States dedicated to the treatment of not only nervous and mental disorders but alcohol and opium addiction as well. It occupied forty acres with four two-story cottages, an amusement hall with a billiard hall in the basement, a flower conservatory, several physical plant buildings, an icehouse, and a station for the Cincinnati Northwestern railroad. Its administration building was once home to the Ohio Female College, which was founded in 1852. The property remained a sanatorium until 1956, when it became the Emerson A. North Hospital. Today the property houses the Cincinnati Children's College Hill Campus, a hospital treating children and adolescents suffering from chronic mental illness and impaired functioning.[16]

## ORPHEUS EVERTS

The fourth son of a beloved Quaker physician named Sylvanus Everts, Orpheus possessed a mechanical and architectural aptitude that he hoped to develop. His father opposed that plan and instead directed his son to study medicine, insisting that his son accompany him on his community rounds. Won over to his father's mission, the younger Everts took up the formal pursuit of medicine in 1843 and became one of a handful of students accepted to Franklin Medical College, the first medical school in Illinois, which lasted only seven years. There he studied under its director, a famous homeopathic physician named George Washington Richards, later also to become Everts's father-in-law.

In 1849–1850, Orpheus Everts became professor of chemistry and pharmacy in the College of the Physicians and Surgeons of the Upper Mississippi at Davenport, Iowa. In 1852 he relinquished his medical practice in favor of accepting a position as editor of a weekly Democratic partisan journal in Laporte. In 1856 he was chosen Democratic elector from the state and cast an electoral vote for James Buchanan for president.[17] He also studied law and was admitted to the bar in 1860. When the Civil War began he resumed his medical profession, became surgeon of the Twentieth Regiment Indiana Volunteers, and was present at all but two of the battles of the Army of the Potomac. After the war he devoted his attention to psychiatry and diseases of the nervous system.

In 1868, Everts was appointed superintendent of the Indiana Hospital for the Insane (later known as Central State), where for the next eleven years he supervised care of the mentally ill and patients diagnosed criminally insane.

In addition to practicing medicine Everts focused on forensics and hospital reform in regard to long-standing patterns of abuse of mentally ill patients. Prior to his tenure at Indiana Hospital, separate facilities for women at the hospital had been nonexistent. Everts pioneered the development of a female department that for the first time housed female patients separately, thus ensuring a measure of privacy and minimizing risk of abuse or assault.

Everts's national recognition as an alienist (forensic psychiatrist) delivered him into prominent legal cases where the question of an accused's sanity was at issue, the most famous of which involved Charles Guiteau, President James A. Garfield's assassin. Together with Selden Talcott and Samuel Worcester, Everts held that Guiteau was sane, testifying that "he had never heard of an insane man denying his act [as Guiteau had done] after it was committed."[18]

## GEORGE WASHINGTON RICHARDS

Orpheus Everts's father-in-law, Dr. George Richards, had graduated from the College of Physicians and Surgeons, New York in 1853. He applied for a position in the New York State Emigrant Hospital, Ward's Island, and received the appointment of assistant house physician, in which he acquitted himself so efficiently that in three months he was offered the primary position of house physician. During his eighteen months with the hospital, nearly eighteen thousand patients were treated.

Dr. Richards toured hospitals in London, Dublin, and Paris and then returned to New York City, where he joined the medical staff of the Hewitt Dispensary. There, over the course of fifteen months during which twenty thousand patients were seen at the dispensary, he began to experiment with homeopathic remedies for chronic skin dis-

dence proving something works as intended; for example, a medical device. The problem arises when we erroneously conclude that something doesn't work or doesn't exist simply because there is no available evidence to support it. This phrase, "There is no evidence to support that," is sometimes used by scientists and journalists in a disingenuous way. When the public hears that phrase, they assume the thing has been investigated and no evidence was found to support it, when in fact, what is usually meant is that the thing has *not been investigated.* So why not just say that? It is misleading and is constantly used to knock down anything not accepted by scientific materialism. Moreover, usually the lack of investigation is not typically due to lack of interest—it is usually because of lack of funding. The majority of science funding in the United States comes from the federal government. The research agendas of most research scientists at academic institutions across the country are determined by what the scientist believes will get funding. Further, federal legislation drives the themes of research for periods of time. For example, after many military personnel returned home from the long wars in the Middle East, an impressive amount of legislation and money was put toward research for traumatic brain injury (TBI), and for post-traumatic stress disorder (PTSD). A TBI is an injury that disrupts normal brain function, and PTSD is a disorder with a constellation of symptoms that develops in some people who have experienced a terrifying and traumatic event. Scientists then scrambled to find a way to frame their research as falling under these themes. Research funding for other topics can come from private foundations. However those funding streams are driven by the personal interests of the wealthy individuals who established the foundations. So please think of this when you hear someone throwing around the word "evidence-based." It would be really nice to have enough money for researchers to investigate anything they wanted and all the interesting questions in the Universe, but in reality, research agendas, and thus evidence and data, are dictated by money, the interests of the government, and wealthy individuals.

I want to take this one step further: What if there are things that can't be measured or explained by the scientific method itself? By deeming the scientific method the *only* important way to measure and understand the world around us, we are inherently saying that if something exists in the Universe that can't be measured by this method, then it is not important or worth knowing. There is a contradiction between believing that we only know for certain what we can measure and observe and the fact that we are using our brains to measure and observe. We know that both physics and quantum physics are true, but we can't reconcile them, and yet we persist in declaring that the scientific method is *the* method.

The limitation of the scientific method is something I encountered on my journey that helped me accept personal proof in addition to scientific proof, and it is also the reason consciousness itself is so hard to study. *There are just some things about the human experience that are hard to quantify and that aren't replicable.* Science can't measure those experiences, and they are usually delegated to the humanities—but then there is no communication between the humanities and science when developing theories about the Universe. We don't experience life in two dimensions, with separate scientific and humanities experiences; it's just one life experience. We need to include both the sciences and the humanities in constructing theories of this stunning, horrid, blissful, cruel thing we call life.

## A MEANINGFUL AND MYSTICAL UNIVERSE

Had I stumbled across all of this information years ago while I was still in graduate school, or even when I had just graduated, I don't think I would have ever written this book. The series of life events that unfolded for me—the power of my mother's readings and predictions and an existential crisis—were all needed to open me up to new modes of thinking. Maybe it all happened in "divine timing," as the intuitives say.

Understanding that consciousness could be the foundation of the Universe reframed my thinking in such a way that unexplained phenomena did not seem extraordinary any longer. It all seemed really simple, actually, and not a big deal. Based on scientific and personal proof,

I now thought it possible that our souls/consciousness reincarnate, carry karma, and evolve by learning lessons. I took this spiritual framework for a test drive and was dazzled at the way it reshaped my interaction with life. When I moved outside the scientific literature into the suggested reading from "the people who know," I learned that the Greeks used the word *Cosmos* to describe the Universe as an orderly system. This is an ancient idea found in most cultures across the world since the beginning of the emergence of humanity. At the confluence of science and spirituality, a new worldview emerged for me: The Universe has meaning and there exists a spiritual and mystical dimension to life. Believing that we are interwoven with the Cosmos and that there is no true distinction between mind and matter, outside and inside, or you and me, has actually been the foundation of reality longer than it hasn't.

# 16

## Pulling Back the Curtain

### Science Is Not Enough

We need more than just science to understand the Cosmos and human experience. I hope there is no doubt about how much I love the scientific method—I did cite scientific research extensively throughout this book! But like anything else, it has its limitations. I discussed a few in the previous chapter, such as how funding drives research topics and not everything about human experience can be measured by the scientific method. Let's pull the curtain back even farther and dig in a bit more by examining scientific assumptions and politics.

## SCIENCE AND THE ACADEMY

By the time I left graduate school I knew that science, and we as a society, most definitely did not have all the answers (although, as I have already mentioned, I was an inductee into the Science Cult and a true believer). When a science experiment is wrapped up, published, and presented to the public, we usually have to summarize the findings in a neat and tidy way that the ordinary public can understand. In actuality, though, biological systems and the natural world are incredibly complex systems that have multiple overlapping and dependent variables. We design studies to the best of our ability to isolate variables so that we can examine causes and effects. We have advanced statistical methods to ascertain the certainty of what we have observed in the experiments, but our statistical thresholds are somewhat arbitrary, and we can sometimes leave unexplained variance within our results in the dust. For each decision made in an experiment, there were plenty of different options to choose from. That means that there are many branch points in the design and analysis of scientific studies, and if you had made a different decision along the way, the results of the study could have turned out completely differently—and they often do, contributing to the "replication crisis" I mentioned earlier.

While it is true that we have good reasons for making the decisions that we do in experiments most of the time, I want to highlight that a lot of the decisions are based on assumptions. In neuroscience in particular, we *assume* that personality traits can be accurately captured and classified by surveys. We *assume* that blood flow in a particular part of the brain indicates that the brain is working in that area and is correlated with behavior. We *assume* that brains across a population are similar enough that we can generalize findings. We *assume* researchers are independent, objective, unbiased components of an experiment who have no effect on the outcome of the experiment. And of course, and this one is important, we *assume* consciousness is produced by the brain. In scientific materialism, as already mentioned, we assume that the physical world is independent of our perceptions, that physical laws can be discovered and described, and that these laws are constant throughout the Cosmos. I make this point because, in order for our results to be accurate, all of those assumptions that we make need to be true.

I go into detail here to convey the complexity of performing scientific research. To be clear, the scientific method is an exceptional tool for investigating and expanding our understanding of the Cosmos. There are many things we learn by using the scientific method, and there are many practical applications of science. Science has aided humanity in finally understanding cause and effect, which has propelled our advancements in medicine and technology, and humans are, albeit arguably, better off now than in centuries before. I'm grateful for the advancement every single morning when I wake up to an automatically ready cup of coffee and an Instagram inbox full of cute animal videos to watch from my friends. Using the pandemic as another example, I appreciate that technology enabled communication during our "two weeks to flatten the curve" that turned into a year-long quarantine. It was scientific progress that provided many beneficial treatments for diseases. Again, I have and will always have profound respect for the scientific process and the advancements it has brought us. Despite this, if any of our assumptions about the Cosmos are wrong—such as that time flows in one direction and that we are independent observers of reality—which they appear to be according to quantum physics—then the models need to be updated.

From a place of appreciation for science and what it has done for humanity, I am going to pull the curtain back a bit farther, because after having gone through this journey I find a tad bit comical the pedestal that science is held upon, especially having been exposed for so long to the incredibly narrow, petty, and infantile reality of the academic scientific world. Reputations and careers are sustained by publishing papers—for which researchers are not compensated—and the sentiment is captured perfectly by the popular phrase "publish or perish." Publications—the currency of a scientist's livelihood—are peer reviewed by scientific competitors (yes, those exist). Can you imagine a venture fund consulting a CEO from a competitor company to review your product (like Nike reviewing Adidas) and making a recommendation on an investment?

The system rewards incremental innovation and staying in line—not earth-shattering, unorthodox, contrarian thinking. Max Planck captured the sentiment well, saying, "Science advances one funeral at a time." We are so narrowly trained and *specialized* that, even within the field of neuroscience, an experimenter studying individual neurons may not even know the different lobes of the human brain! They are brilliant, beautiful, earnest people trapped in a broken system.

So despite science being invaluable, many fundamental limitations and practical constraints prevent it from being the only method capable of helping us understand the Cosmos and human experience. Mainstream science encourages curiosity and open thinking, but you know, not *too* open, not *too* curious.

# 17

# Moving Toward a
# Meaningful Cosmos

*Our psyche is set up in accord with the structure of the universe,
and what happens in the macrocosm likewise happens in the
infinitesimal and most subjective reaches of the psyche.*

C. G. JUNG

Continuing to explore other fields of knowledge, I came to realize that although the modern Western worldview is quite dominant in the present day, it has only existed for a sliver of human existence. Many of its foundational philosophies were birthed during the Scientific Revolution and the Age of Enlightenment. Before those two movements, religion provided an understanding of the world and, by providing a reason for existence, supplied meaning to life. From the rational and physicalist beliefs of the Enlightenment, the Cosmos eventually came to be viewed as inherently random and meaningless. As scientific advancements provided increasing control over nature, and previous mysteries of the world became explainable, a deep reverence for science, and the skepticism we see exhibited by scientific materialism, emerged. It was believed that scientific progress was limitless and, eventually, everything could be explained by scientific methods.

It's true we have seen miraculous progress, but it's also true that *many many* things in the world remain mysterious, and instead of trying to explore these mysteries, scientific materialism has decided to ignore them. The benefits of the West's view of the world have come at significant costs, some being manifested as modern-day society's increased existential and mental health crises. Let's look at some of the differences between worldviews and how the Western worldview may not be working out for us as hoped, after all.

## WESTERN VS. ANIMA MUNDI WORLDVIEWS

The boundary between self and other, subject and object, and human and nature are different between the modern Western worldview and the holistic and ecological worldview characteristic of traditional indigenous cultures (as well as the ancient Greeks, medieval scholastics, Renaissance humanists, and many more). In the latter worldview, the entire world and Cosmos are viewed as having a soul, an anima mundi. For simplicity, I will refer to this as the anima mundi worldview. Everything—humans, plants, animals, the Earth, stars, planets—are connected in a living matrix that is naturally embedded with meaning. These cultures find meaning in everything, including the patterns of weather, the activity of animals, and the movement of stars. To them, the world is intelligent, intentional, spiritual, meaningful, alive, and purposeful, and it communicates through symbols and archetypes. The human psyche is viewed as part of the Cosmos, and the Cosmos is part of the human psyche, because we are a microcosm of the macrocosm (Tarnas 2006). In this system, it is believed humans can access this intelligent matrix with their own subconscious minds through altered states of consciousness that can be achieved through dance, chanting, substances, and other methods. Typically, individuals will be selected and trained in these spiritual and mystical practices to heal, perform divination, or control events, such as in shamanism. Cultures that subscribe to the anima mundi worldview are mindful of balance with nature because they believe they are intimately and divinely connected to it.

This worldview is in sharp contrast to the modern Western worldview that sees humankind as completely separate from its surroundings; in other words, as a subject separate from objects, including all living and nonliving things. Meaning is created solely from the human mind and should not be projected onto the external world or the Cosmos, which are inherently random, mechanistic, and purposeless. With this ideology and its advancement in science, humans have aimed to control and dominate nature as a resource to be owned and utilized for the benefit of humankind. This patriarchal worldview prioritizes rationality, logic, reason, productivity, individuality, hierarchies, and domination over emotion, intuition, compassion, equality, sustainability, and partnership. Anything not aligned with the tenets is denigrated.

The thing is, though, as depth psychologist Richard Tarnas (2006) puts it, the anima mundi ". . . cosmos was universally *experienced*, for countless millennia, as tangibly self-evidently alive and awake—pervasively intentional and responsive, informed by ubiquitous spiritual presences, animated throughout by archetypal forces and intelligible meanings."

## IT'S NOT WORKING OUT

There are countless ways the modern Western worldview has failed us, and I will expand on a few here that most pertain to spiritual and mystical experiences. In particular, I'll look at how the ideology has harmed us as an integrated society trying to understand life, as well as on an individual existential level.

The Western worldview, naturally, asserts itself as the dominant view of the world and condescendingly refers to other types of thinking or ways of being that challenge its foundational ideas as irrational, primitive, inferior, or undeveloped. It excludes countering narratives from mainstream culture with derision, makes those who are different feel their ideas and cultures are wrong, and causes pressure for conformity. Insisting and asserting that the Western worldview is the best and only respectable one is one way the West has demeaned and marginalized all other cultures and peoples. Women, too, have long been sidelined by the patriarchal West. Think of women being stereotyped as having greater intuition, an internal state that operates independently of reason. Is it a mere coincidence that we are then trained to be untrustworthy of that intuition (Rosenbaum 2011; Barušs and Mossbridge 2017)? The real kicker, though, is that scientific evidence shows that some of the tenets that we celebrate from the Age of Enlightenment are actually much more complicated than is generally believed, such as the finding that relying on unconscious processing of information, or intuition, can be advantageous in certain circumstances, such as decision making (Dijksterhuis et al. 2006; Voss, Lucas, and Paller 2012; Voss, Baym, and Paller 2008). Yet still, belief in things that the West deems impossible are referred to derogatorily as irrational, delusional, crazy, and magical thinking, despite the fact that the people usually espousing such beliefs are none of those things.

The experience of entire groups of people, such as those who experience subtle energy and unexplained phenomena, is also discounted. But we saw from the Cardeña (2018) meta-analysis that there is scientific evidence; and we can even see one possible mechanism for transcendental experience and subtle energy perception from the accounts from neuroscientist Dr. Bolte Taylor, whose brain's left hemisphere, the one responsible for reasoning, essentially went off-line after a stroke. She showed us that the right hemisphere does perceive subtle energy dynamics in a way that our left hemisphere does not.

She writes:

> I hope your level of discomfort about such things as energy dynamics and intuition has decreased as you have increased your understanding about the fundamental differences in the way our two hemispheres collaborate to create our single perception of reality. . . . Our right hemisphere is designed to perceive and decipher the subtle energy dynamics we perceive intuitively. Since the stroke, I steer my life almost entirely by paying attention to how people, places, and things feel to me energetically.

She also writes:

> Our right brain perceives the big picture and recognizes that everything around us, about us, among us, and within us is made up of energy particles that are woven together into a universal tapestry. Since everything is connected, there is an intimate relationship between the atomic space around and within me, and the atomic space around and within you—regardless of where we are.

The power that drives our nervous system and keeps our heart beating is just energy. Our senses receive energy signals that our brains translate. If you ever need a reminder, think of how humans appear on infrared cameras. Is it, then, still woo-woo to think that some people's brains are wired in such a way that the subtle energy detection ability of the right hemisphere is enhanced, as it was for Dr. Bolte Taylor following her stroke? It's entirely possible.

Terrence McKenna (1992), an ethnobotanist, wrote that when he visited the Amazon, he carried the Western world's assumptions that science could prove everything and that belief in magic, divination, or spiritual healing, the kind performed by Amazonian shamans, was naive. But after a few psychedelic trips, he wrote, "I was initially appalled at what I found: the world of shamanism, of allies, shape shifting, and magical attack are far more real than the constructs of science can ever be, because these spirit ancestors and their other world can be seen and felt, they can be known, in the nonordinary reality."

McKenna also believed that our disconnection from our unconscious minds and the anima mundi, living matrix, nature, and spiritual dimension—and the zero-point field?—have propelled humanity into the crisis of meaningless existence in which it now finds itself. I now happen to agree. Our society would have us believe we are birthed into an uncaring, indifferent world and we should nurture our sense of abandonment ourselves. A search is undertaken by the modern person to fill the missing hole, but they find nothing but anguish, frustration, shallow moments of joy, disappointment, and deep unfulfillment. No wonder the United States has a mental health crisis in which one in five Americans lives with a mental health condition (according to the National Alliance on Mental Illness), and there exists an alarming shortage of behavioral health practitioners. We can't find the missing pieces of ourselves, or our connection to the sacred, in a new Xbox, a Balenciaga gown, or a larger house.

I would include scientists in this group of people afflicted by mental health conditions. Let's even assume momentarily that the evolutionary theories are true about religious and spiritual belief systems having evolved to protect humans from the suffering of life by building meaning into events. Why do skeptics, believing they are upholding Western values, try so hard to squash that if it has a purported evolutionary purpose? Will we disadvantage the species in some way by doing so? As we saw earlier, scientists are split down the middle in whether they believe in a higher power, but those who do believe have reported feeling uncomfortable expressing their views to their colleagues. Why are we so inauthentic? Are we surprised about the high rates of mental health issues when scientists' livelihood requires them to think there is no meaning behind life? On the one hand, the scientific world condescendingly argues that stories of religion and spirituality are mechanisms of comfort and coping to help make it through the hellish existence of human life on Earth, and then we deprive scientists of having that comfort at the fear of ostracism and stigma? I wish I had known that before I went to graduate school!

I also believe the pushback on ideas, phenomena, or modalities that are not aligned with Western values is justified by the patriarchy with a narrative of "protection," especially when it comes to medicine and healing—which is a whole nother can of worms. Usually when people say something doesn't have evidence, they mean it could actually harm you. Those fears are not unjustified. I am keenly aware that belief can sometimes move people away from science in dangerous ways. Modern science and medicine have also, however, failed us in some ways. For physical and mental healing, in particular, I believe Western medicine comes up short. But rather than admit its weaknesses, we see the suppression of decentralized, alternate, and unconventional ideas with arrogance through patriarchal and hierarchical structures. Since the Western worldview prioritizes external, objective data, patients can struggle to be heard by their health care practitioners—a well-known consequence of this being the historic dismissal of the subjective experiences of women patients in Western medicine. Patients may feel judged by their health care practitioners when disclosing the use of healing remedies from their own non-Western cultures. I think people should be supported in seeking all healing modalities, especially when Western medicine has failed them. While protection from harm is important, shouldn't there also be room in health care for compassion, understanding, and inclusivity? As we saw from the meta-analysis of the noncontact healing studies, energy medicine has some budding scientific support. It also has significant anecdotal personal support from countless individuals, which may not be enough for statistically minded fields but could mean everything for a person in pain.

In summary, certain aspects of the Western worldview are not working for us, such as prioritizing reason and empirical evidence over intuition and personal experience, thereby denying the mystical and spiritual aspects of the world and that the world has meaning. The effects are seen in the way people and groups with different perspectives feel marginalized and inferior; this is creating a disintegrated society, as well as the existential and mental health crises of our society and limitations to the ways we heal.

## MOVING FORWARD

I didn't write this book to just complain about my existential crisis and transformation. I really believe there is great potential in broadening our worldview by incorporating the evidence of spiritual and unexplained phenomena, because it hints at a radiantly interlaced reality where we are more supported than we think. Here are some implications I see for moving forward.

## IMPLICATIONS FOR HEALING

What most caught my attention from the past life regression literature, and then again later in the psychedelic work, was the surprising and extensive mental and physical healing that resulted from the practice. This is *the* most important implication, in my opinion. Not only did the extensive literature on altered states of consciousness reveal effective resolution of chronic mental and physical issues, but I also personally experienced the dramatic healing effects. As mentioned above, Western medicine, psychiatry, and psychology leave much to be desired, and is it any wonder when they are using incomplete models of the Cosmos derived from only one worldview? I am grateful that there are a number of formally trained health practitioners recognizing this problem and working to incorporate more healing modalities to address trauma, such as Drs. Dan Siegel, Gabor Maté, Peter Levine, and Bessel Van der Kolk. But we need much more than a small cohort of broad-minded thinkers. Our society is plagued with mental health issues and unresolved trauma, and we take our issues out into the world with us. Instead of focusing on healing ourselves—arguably the most important thing one can do—our society is focused on acquiring material success. It's time to change that. It's time to combine the scientific accomplishments since the Enlightenment, the developments in psychology from the past 150 years, and other worldviews in addition to the West's to heal ourselves and find purpose.

## IMPLICATIONS FOR SCIENCE

Science needs to cross into interdisciplinary territory to tackle the gigantic questions of fully comprehending the Cosmos and human experience—and I mean *way* across the aisle. All scientists need to seek knowledge from other disciplines to help place scientific materialism into a larger human historic context. Many subfields of the humanities, such as anthropology, the history of non-Western cultures, and ethnobotany, to name just a few, can potentially provide new ways of thinking about systems and cycles of nature. Philosophy can help supply the subjective component of understanding consciousness that science cannot address. While neuroscience has been enormously informative about the underlying biological mechanisms of behavior, especially in animal studies, clinical psychology can provide insight into what actually truly works on shaping human behavior and healing trauma and interpersonal issues in the real world, as opposed to in the lab. In fact, while the majority of psychedelic research of the current day has come from neuroscience labs, the initial extensive, comprehensive, and groundbreaking work of using psychedelics for personal healing has come from transpersonal psychology. If you really want to have your mind blown, read anything written by Stanislav Grof, one of the founders of transpersonal psychology. Also, depth psychology, particularly Carl Jung's work, provides unique observations and theories about synchronicities and how the human psyche is inextricably linked to the Cosmos.

Now that we have scientific and philosophical models that help explain spiritual and mystical experiences, as well as the experiences of intuitives, mediums, and energy healers, would it be too wild to suggest that we also include metaphysics in the conversation? Maybe we should listen more closely to people who claim to be sensitive to subtle energy because their descriptions of how things work might lead us to more answers? For example, when reviewing the neuroscientific findings earlier, I found descriptions of the new brain metric, CHD, that showed a spectrum of consciousness from anesthesia up to psychedelics with increasing frequency harmonics. When reading the finding, I immediately thought about how people who subscribe to New Age thought always seem to be talking about keeping your vibrations high to access the higher levels of consciousness, and how that enables you to be in flow with the Universe. Maybe that kind of elevated state truly does allow you to connect to the zero-point field better (I can't believe I'm saying this). Of course, this is a huge jump, and I'm just using this example to demonstrate how the phenomenological experiences of unexplained phenomena could be useful in moving forward with scientific theory. As yet another example, Keppler suggested measuring phase transitions in the brain with photons. Maybe that's why intuitives and mediums use the words "light energy" when describing mystical things. I used to roll my eyes at those words, but now I have seen an actual scientific model proposing such a thing in a peer-reviewed scientific journal. I know this is a blasphemous suggestion, and I'm imagining some scientists recoiling at the thought of respectfully engaging with spiritual or metaphysical people. I'd tell them what many of the intuitives I went to see (embarrassingly) told me: *Get off your high horse.* There's already a bit of progress with labs, like the COPE Project at Yale, taking seriously the claims of individuals that see and hear more things than others (i.e., intuitives, mediums, mystics, and those with visual and auditory "hallucinations") and investigating the differences between these individuals, who are capable of living normal and healthy lives, and those with serious mental illness who are not. But imagine what else we can learn!

If we take the model of cosmopsychism, as just one example, and ask whether mental illness is perhaps a broken connection with the zero-point field, as Keppler ponders, we can study how this might be solved with a new technology or therapeutic practice. Or perhaps we could identify the override function from savants and terminal lucidity and extend the application to TBI, stroke, and dementia patients. Maybe by using newly developed methods of more easily tapping into the zero-point field we will find greater insight into the inner working of the Universe, providing inspiration for new scientific breakthroughs. The possibilities are endless. It's not science fiction; I believe it could be the future of science.

It is important to continue doing traditional science research because it does have benefits, but it is also imperative that we invest in research supporting models other than scientific materialism to begin filling the holes in our incomplete model. Ultimately, whether consilience between the fields is obtainable is open to debate, but it is imperative that we work as though it is.

One more thing: If you are a scientist reading this and have never experienced anything mystical or spiritual, I want to invite you to try. Is meditation too demanding? Get a metaphysical reading of any kind, whether energy or intuitive or astrological or whatever. If you approach it with an open mind, you just might be surprised. I'm not promising you will be astonished because, as I have outlined in this book, there are many unknown factors that influence these interactions. But what do you have to lose? Thirty minutes of your time? Or maybe an hour and a half of your time if you get three different readings (which I recommend) to really get a good sample. You might come away with a completely new understanding of one (common) type of human experience.

## IMPLICATIONS FOR SPIRITUALITY

I was vehemently anti-spiritual until my worldview failed me to the point that I wished I didn't exist. Although I was flirting with the idea that some kind of meaning structured the Cosmos by getting intuitive readings, I didn't use any spiritual framework to rethink my perspective of life until I was repeatedly confronted with the reincarnation and karma spiritual framework, and especially from clinical psychology and psychiatry. Because my mind works best with mechanisms, the scientific evidence for psi and the consciousness theories of the Cosmos helped bridge personal experience with spirituality. I am now comfortable accepting that I believe that meaning creates the Cosmos and that there is indeed a spiritual and mystical component. For me, the idea of a meaningful Cosmos immediately reduced my suffering. Adding on the framework of reincarnation, karma, and soul lessons was a bonus, creating a narrative for understanding my life's events.

If this is not our one and only life, and we truly carry karma over into the next ones, shouldn't we be behaving better? I know that for me, personally, reading all this material has changed the way I think about life and the way I behave. I am definitely not perfect by any means, but I try to be more cognizant of the way I think about situations, how I treat people, and how consciously I make decisions that align with my values. As cliché as it sounds, I try to lead with love and understanding. I fail a ton, but I try. That's why it's called a spiritual *practice*. We can start working together more effectively as a global population, say to address social justice and climate change issues, by seeing the truth: that we are one interconnected consciousness. Let's take seriously the results of the Global Consciousness Project that showed, when mass consciousness and attention were sharply focused on one event, random number generators behaved nonrandomly. As we improve our inner worlds, we also can improve the outer world. Feeling that deep interconnectedness among us can help shift our attention from the differences between us to the common issues that face us all, such as social justice, climate change, and the economy.

Personal experiential proof is important, too. If 5% of the human population experienced something like, say, their eyes turning purple for ten seconds every time they reached their max heart rate, but a study to quantify and document the effect was never conducted, would that mean the effect doesn't exist? Of course not. The purple eye syndrome would be very real for the 5% of people who experience it, and it shouldn't be discounted. Unfortunately, Western culture has made us question our own experiences, but they're important, too!

In summary, the implications range from poetic to practical. I brought you on my long journey in this book because trying to tie together unexplained phenomena, spirituality, science, and altered states of consciousness healing techniques at the outset would have been a challenge, not only to understand, but to accept—for both you and me! I hope I have laid a groundwork that more easily shows the connections and implications of these interrelated topics. If you choose to launch a personal exploration, you can start your own journey. I would even go so far as to say, after my own journey into the topic, that you might try to unbind your consciousness, soar through the oceanic Cosmos, touch the divine, and bring back a bit of magic to your everyday life. You might find a piece of yourself that you didn't know had been hiding. As a society, we should support internal flights through altered states of consciousness because of the dramatic healing that can arise. I also hope we can bridge fields of knowledge to exponentially advance our understanding of the Cosmos and, as a natural consequence, be more inclusive of the experiences and beliefs of others, because, even if it's not always obvious, we are one splendid labyrinth of glittering consciousness.

# 18

# Sometimes Things Need to Die

*You are not a drop in the ocean. You are the entire ocean in a drop.*

RUMI

The death of your ego, your old life, your old self happens one thousand times—being only slightly less painful each passing. Similarly, healing happens bit by bit, one thousand more times.

As I said in the preface, I wished this had never happened and that I never had to write this book. In time, though, I have come to see this experience as a gift. Hopefully, this happens eventually for all of us with all experiences, but this shift in perspective began emerging for me unexpectedly from an interview I heard of Stephen Colbert by Anderson Cooper (Cooper 2019). Anderson Cooper had just lost his beloved mother, Gloria Vanderbilt, and asked Stephen Colbert, who lost his father and two brothers in a plane crash when he was ten years old, about how he previously had said that he had come to learn to "love the thing that I most wish had not happened." The rest of the exchange is below:

"You went on to say, 'What punishments of God are not gifts?' Do you really believe that?" Cooper asked.

"Yes," Colbert said. "It's a gift to exist and with existence comes suffering. There's no escaping that. What do you get from loss? You get awareness of other people's loss, which allows you to connect with that other person, which allows you to love more deeply and to understand what it's like to be a human being, if it's true that all humans suffer."

One reason I decided to write this book is that the journey was so mentally difficult for me—with so much belief and disbelief and uncertainty and revisiting of evidence. I saw firsthand within myself what it took to overthrow, or adjust, a belief system—even when faced with compelling evidence from decades of research from many labs, scientists, and other scholars. It was *damn* hard. My old beliefs went kicking and screaming, leaving scars in their wake. As my old beliefs tore away from me, they wrapped their tendrils around some of my self-illusions and forced me to *very reluctantly* face myself. Then I saw that it wasn't the beliefs I was attached to. It was the self-worth I thought I could earn through the beliefs.

My own existential crisis truly was a gift because it helped me to understand the broader range of human emotions, like despair and intense, unrelenting anger. I hope it has made me a more understanding and compassionate person. The image that comes to mind when I think of the crisis is a shattered mirror. Watching the broken pieces come back together in slow-motion rewind through my healing efforts has been surprisingly gratifying.

As for my intellectual journey, years of scientific training were no joke. The concepts and skepticism were so deeply ingrained in me that, no matter the vigor with which I tried to erase them, there still remained remnants of the pencil marks on the page. There was a lasting impression that continuously resurfaced, just when I thought I found new beliefs or turned the page. The new beliefs could, it seemed, so easily be overturned or, in the least, have a pin put in them for further consideration. For a return look. For a repeat tumble through the skepticism dryer. What would it take to finally accept a new belief system? Or was the identity so deeply ingrained that it wasn't possible?

It's just an identity, though. An ethereal concept. Something solid but ever changing, and something that can (apparently) cause a lot of inner turmoil. Or it's the attachment to the identity that causes the suffering. In thinking about this, it occurred to me that I'd have to grieve for my former self in some way to really accept the new version of myself that is open to ideas that are not yet accepted by scientific materialism. This book is part of that grieving process. In the end it was such a lovely gift to become more open minded to alternative views of the world, where I am the Cosmos and the Cosmos is me. Personal transformation is difficult because of our deep-seated identities and embodied beliefs, but it is possible to transform with hard work, surrendering, and asking, "What if I'm wrong?" Through my transformation, I eventually realized that I was only losing the identity of the person I *thought I should be*. One way I think about the process is as death and rebirth. When one identity dies, I let go, grieve, and let something new come in; this allows for a new identity to be born. Or I think of it as an unearthing of additional parts of myself. Each newly discovered part fuses with the previous parts to form a new whole, a new identity. Through it all, we can have compassion for ourselves for the experience. I have been intensely and thoroughly humbled in my ego's death and rebirth, and I hope to keep this humility with me as I continue moving through this life.

In reading esoteric texts, I found elegant knowledge and symbolism for the cycles of life: birth and death, light and dark, activity and rest, beginnings and endings, happiness and sadness, joy and despair. An understanding that sometimes things need to die to be replaced by better things could alleviate fear of transformation and help us all face ourselves.

At the beginning of this journey, I could not see what was causing my personal darkness, my dark night. A broken heart? Dissatisfaction with my career? That I didn't have a $20 million house in Bel Air? It turns out it was something far broader: my worldview. Living without meaning and purpose in a random, dead Universe was not working out for me, but I never would have come to this understanding by myself. I was lucky to have a series of coincidences lead me to spiritual exploration and self-actualization, which I now believe are parts of the purpose of life.

I now consider myself a spiritual scientist, and it fills me with indescribable light and joy to say that. It was, after all, a hard-earned destination. Finally, a semblance of peace has floated into my day-to-day existence. It's not that life got easier; it's just that my perspective changed. I still find myself having all the human trappings of desiring things, wanting specific outcomes, and reaching for some sort of control, but I practice letting go whenever I can. Believing that things happen for a reason and that maybe—*just maybe*—I chose these specific challenges for myself prior to this lifetime helps me take a step back, calm down, and not see myself as a victim of life. Honestly, whether I ever find out if the spiritual framework is true or not, I wouldn't trade this journey for anything.

One of my best friends told me that the ultimate test of my evolution would be my answer to the question, "Do you believe in God?" After a lifetime of flipping the bird to the word "God," it was admittedly hard to accept any kind of intelligence behind the Universe. That is the concept with which I have the most trouble. Reading the literature from physics and cosmology, though, and seeing that the odds of the emergence of the Universe and life were so slim that even physicists and cosmologists are amazed, did make me pause. Wondering whether we would ever be able to prove such a thing, it occurred to me that if there truly was an intelligence who was orchestrating things, then it would in no way be obligated to bow to our scientific method. Heck, if I were the intelligence behind everything and I was watching my human babies try to measure me, catch me, prove me, I would *most definitely* have some fun with it!

I don't know as a definitive fact that the spiritual framework involving soul lessons, karma, and reincarnation is true, but I can say that there is compelling scientific and personal evidence, and I can *choose* to believe it. Anything is possible! It is definitely worth investigating.

As for research into unexplained phenomena, if we hold it to the same standard as other fields of science, the results are very strongly in support of its existence. Personally, I have also had far too many out-of-this-world accurate intuitive readings and direct personal experiences to question the phenomena any longer. Sure, there is no *agreed-upon* mechanism. But what's so controversial about that? We don't know how the placebo effect works, either, but we accept that it does. So let's find out, and if everything truly is one field of interconnected consciousness (and that's where I'm leaning right now), then the phenomena are not anomalous at all—they're simply tapping into our broader consciousness.

It was comforting to know that many people had experiences similar to that of mine and my mother's. In fact, I now believe we are the majority, not the minority. The dominance of scientific materialism and rationalism have constituted but a mere few hundred years of human existence, while the idea of being enmeshed with something greater than ourselves, an ensouled and meaningful Universe, has existed and served humans for thousands of years and still exists in many, if not most, (non-Western) cultures around the world. What we have come to readily mock in Western civilization as complete and utter nonsense and magical thinking has been used by humans around the world to guide purposeful, fulfilling lives for millennia. We may yet find that this theory of scientific materialism and the Western worldview that some of us currently use as the foundation of our version of reality does not in fact serve our best interests and can be replaced with something better. What I do know is that our current scientific models are not enough to accommodate my personal experiences—nor those of countless others—and that the evidence for expanded consciousness provides a more likely explanation thus far.

I continue to periodically have intuitive readings, but this is no longer out of desperation or need for control, but rather because they help me with more deeply knowing myself. I find intuitive readings to be healing. Maybe it is because they can actually see so many layers of me and my energy. Maybe it's because I can unburden my heavy heart. Or maybe, like one of the mystics I spoke with suggested, intuitives, psychic mediums, energy healers, and mystics create space for you to heal yourself—because at the end of the day, no one can heal you but you. The signs of a spiritual experience can be subtle, and you have to be cognizant. Also, if you have a brain like mine that is adamant on being kept peace-free, the skepticism floats up to hammer out any magic. I imagine it would take years of belief retraining to rewire those neural circuits of mine, and I am not sure that would even be for the best. A healthy dose of skepticism is necessary for the modern world.

Having said that, I'll tell you the one piece of evidence that knocked me off my feet. Before I had jumped into my interview project and had only begun reading the past life regression literature, I read somewhere that you could ask the Universe or your spirit guides, or whatever you believed in, for a sign. I had sort of been trying this off and on, but I was choosing signs that were not that specific, and most of the time I would forget what sign I had even chosen. Since I was unreliable, one day I thought I would try one last time and put the responsibility on the Universe by asking it for a sign so big that even I couldn't miss, meaning that it couldn't be something like a butterfly or a bird. It had to be something significant to me, but since I was bad at choosing signs, I left it up to the Universe as to what that should be. Two nights later I was in an Uber going to meet my friends to celebrate a birthday. On the way to the restaurant one of them called me and asked how far away I was from the restaurant. I told her I was about five minutes away and asked why. She said, "You are not going to believe who is here! CHELSEA HANDLER!" I got chills from head to toe. Are. You. Kidding. Me?!?!?! I knew this was my sign.

I got to the restaurant, and there she was in all her vintage-tee-wearing glory with family and friends eating dinner. It was none other than the woman whose podcast interview with Laura Lynne Jackson had led me to Brian Weiss's book and, ultimately, this whole crazy ride! She also so deeply inspired me with her own transformation story and gave me strength to embrace the change. The Universe could not have possibly chosen a more meaningful sign for me, and I was in awe—but also still a bit intimidated by the Universe! I felt like I was in conversation with the Universe, and I was tingling. I did not want to bother

Chelsea while she was at dinner, but as we left the restaurant at the same time, I did make sure to tell her that I loved her book and podcast. Yes, it is LA, and we run into celebrities now and again, as I'm sure the skeptics would like to point out. But it certainly isn't daily, and I have never seen her before or since. The meaningfulness of that night still gives me goose bumps. We may never be able to prove whether the meaning we construct from personal events like the one I had that night are a gift from the Universe or spirit world, or rather just internally generated from my coincidence-detector brain—but it doesn't change the fact that meaning existed in that moment, and I was reminded of how the Universe could sparkle for us.

Yes, sparkle *for us*. That means you, too. Because as I came to find in my review of the literature, theories from both physics and philosophy leave a door open for a participatory Universe. If we live in a participatory Universe, it matters how you show up for yourself and for others. Whether you show up with positivity or negativity *matters*. I now try to move through life being more awake, always assessing whether things align with my values, and trying to be conscious. What if our brains seek patterns and meaning because there are patterns and meaning to be found? I liked the way Mark Booth put it in *The Secret History of the World:* "Cicero and Newton were idealists. They experienced life as meaningful, and the cosmos as meant. They believed, then, that something like human qualities, indeed something like human consciousness, is built into the structure of the cosmos."

Now, as I wrap up this book, I am still devouring as much knowledge as I can—and I imagine this will continue until the end of my time. Although this experience started with following what I deemed the only worthy kind of evidence—scientific—into the world of the mysterious, I am now open to all types of knowledge and understand that, to truly begin to grasp the nature of the world and our experience of it, we must reach across and through different fields and types of thought. You will not get the answers from just science, or from any other single field.

How do I decide what to read and study next? I try to take, as my friend Royce says, "inspired action." I follow my intuition and what excites me. I imagine being in one of those long hallways, the type you might find in an old English manor, and moving down past the doors until I feel the pull to enter a doorway.

As of this current moment, I am diving into Western astrology (the full birth chart analysis type, not the popular magazine sun sign horoscopes), which is, again, another field of study I never believed in and that society, on the whole, doesn't bother to understand on a deeper level. The jury is still out for me on the effectiveness of astrology in guiding or understanding the events of life, but I did find it to be profoundly useful as a psychological tool that can elicit many personal insights. Recently, it left me with yet another experience of wonder. I was reading about my lunar phase, which is the phase of the moon under which you were born and which allegedly tells about your soul purpose or mission. My moon phase happens to be a disseminating moon, represented by the archetypes of the pilgrim, teacher, servant, mystic, Virgo type. These archetypes even fit 'old me,' as someone who was asking questions and seeking knowledge. As my life unfolded, these questions became more complex, and that led me to look beyond science and, ultimately, to blend science and spirituality in my own life. Let me explain this in more detail.

Those born under this moon phase purportedly are drawn toward intellectual pursuits of discovering universal truths through experience, but with the ultimate purpose of then disseminating—hence the name of the phase—all the knowledge they have gained in a practical way to society in order for it to be helpful. Another motif associated with this lunar phase is death and rebirth. People born under this lunar phase can come to question the meaning of their lives through the confrontation of suffering and undergo a "spiritual conversion midway through life—a symbolic death and rebirth where they leave their old life behind and completely change direction" (Thurman 2016). I chuckled out loud when I read this description because that has been exactly my experience, as a scientist-turned-spiritual believer, and I hope to share it with others through writing this book in order to be helpful to anyone else who finds themself in a position similar to mine. At least I am in good company, as some examples of other disseminating moons include Ram Dass, Alan Watts, Alan Ginsberg, Aldous Huxley, Albert Einstein, and even the guitarist from my favorite band, The Beatles, George Harrison.

I came to think of my prior self as someone living in a cave (a smart person in a nice, comfortable cave, but limited nonetheless). I thought of (what I am now considering) my life crisis as an earthquake that caused the domed rock of the cave to crack wide open, allowing sunlight to pour in. The cave was nice before, but the shimmering daylight is incomparably exquisite with its illuminating warmth. I never want to step out of the sun again.

From that image of warmth and light, I want to leave you with this: What would you research, read, or begin learning next to further your life experience for the better? I invite you to get personally acquainted with the enchanted and numinous dimensions of life in whatever way you choose! This is your invitation from the Cosmos.

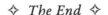

✧ *The End* ✧

# Recommended Reads

## CONSCIOUSNESS

Barušs, Imants, and Julia Mossbridge (2017) *Transcendent Mind: Rethinking the Science of Consciousness*. Washington, D.C.: American Psychological Association.

Dossey, Larry (2014) *One Mind: How Our Individual Mind Is Part of a Greater Consciousness and Why It Matters*. Carlsbad, Calif: Hay House Inc.

Gober, Mark (2018) *An End to Upside Down Thinking*. Hampshire, UK: Waterside Press.

Kelly, Edward F., Adam Crabtree, and Paul Marshall (Eds.) (2015) *Beyond Physicalism: Toward Reconciliation of Science and Spirituality*. Lanham, Md.: Rowman & Littlefield.

Kelly, Edward F., Emily Williams Kelly, Adam Crabtree, Alan Gauld, and Michael Grosso (Eds.) (2007) *Irreducible Mind: Toward a Psychology for the 21st Century*. Lanham, Md.: Rowman & Littlefield.

Kelly, Edward F., and Paul Marshall (Eds.) (2021) *Consciousness Unbound: Liberating Mind from the Tyranny of Materialism*. Lanham, Md.: Rowman & Littlefield.

Kripal, Jeffrey J. (2019) *The Flip: Epiphanies of Mind and the Future of Knowledge*. New York: Bellevue Literary Press.

Sheldrake, Rupert (2018) *Science and Spiritual Practices: Transformative Experiences and Their Effects on Our Bodies, Brains, and Health*. Berkeley, Calif: Counterpoint Press.

Tart, Charles (2009) *The End of Materialism: How Evidence of the Paranormal*

*Is Bringing Science and Spirit Together.* Oakland, Calif: New Harbinger Publications.

## PAST LIFE REGRESSION

Newton, Michael (2010) *Destiny of Souls: New Case Studies of Life Between Lives.* Woodbury, Minn.: Llewellyn Worldwide.
Newton, Michael (1994) *Journey of Souls: Case Studies of Life Between Lives.* Woodbury, Minn.: Llewellyn Publications.
Webber, John (2020) *The Red Chair.* Carlsbad, Calif: Balboa Press.
Weiss, Brian L. (1988) *Many Lives, Many Masters.* New York: Simon & Schuster.
Weiss, Brian L. (1992) *Through Time Into Healing.* New York: Simon & Schuster.
Woolger, Roger J. (1988) *Other Lives, Other Selves: A Jungian Psychotherapist Discovers Past Lives.* New York: Bantam Books.

## SPIRITUALITY

Dass, Ram (1971) *Be Here Now.* New York: Three Rivers Press.
Salzberg, Sharon (1999) *A Heart as Wide as the World: Stories on the Path of Loving Kindness.* Boulder, Colo.: Shambhala Publications.
Satchidananda, S. (1984) *The Yoga Sutras of Patanjali: Translation and Commentary by Sri Swami Satchidananda.* Buckingham, Va.: Integral Yoga Publications.
Singer, Michael A. (2007) *The Untethered Soul: The Journey Beyond Yourself.* Oakland, Calif: New Harbinger Publications.

## PSYCHEDELICS

Fadiman, James (2011) *The Psychedelic Explorer's Guide: Safe, Therapeutic, and Sacred Journeys.* New York: Simon & Schuster.
Leary, Timothy, Ralph Metzner, and Richard Alpert (1964) *The Psychedelic Experience: A Manual Based on the Tibetan Book of the Dead.* New York: University Books.
McKenna, Terence (1999) *Food of the Gods: The Search for the Original Tree of Knowledge: A Radical History of Plants, Drugs and Human Evolution.* New York: Random House.
Pollan, Michael (2019) *How to Change Your Mind: What the New Science of*

*Psychedelics Teaches Us about Consciousness, Dying, Addiction, Depression, and Transcendence.* New York: Penguin Books.

## NEW TO PSI RESEARCH

Carpenter, J. C. (2015) *First Sight: ESP and Parapsychology in Everyday Life.* Lanham, Md.: Rowman & Littlefield.

Dossey, Larry (2014) *One Mind: How Our Individual Mind Is Part of a Greater Consciousness and Why It Matters.* Carlsbad, Calif: Hay House Inc.

Gober, Mark (2018) *An End to Upside Down Thinking.* Hampshire, UK: Waterside Press.

Jacobsen, Annie (2017) *Phenomena: The Secret History of the U.S. Government's Investigations into Extrasensory Perception and Psychokinesis.* New York: Little, Brown and Company.

Kean, Leslie (2017) *Surviving Death: A Journalist Investigates Evidence for an Afterlife.* New York: Crown Archetype.

Radin, Dean (2013) *Supernormal: Science, Yoga, and the Evidence for Extraordinary Psychic Abilities.* La Jolla, Calif.: Deepak Chopra Books.

Targ, Russell (2012) *The Reality of ESP: A Physicist's Proof of Psychic Abilities.* Wheaton, Ill.: Theosophical Publishing House.

## MEDIUMSHIP/PSYCHIC/INTUITIVE

Beischel, Julie (2014) *From the Mouths of Mediums.* Vol. 1: *Experiencing Communication.* Tucson, Ariz.: Windbridge Institute, LLC.

Beischel, Julie (2015) *Investigating Mediums: A Windbridge Institute Collection.* San Francisco: Blurb.

Beischel, Julie (2013) *Meaningful Messages: Making the Most of Your Mediumship Reading.* Tucson, Ariz.: Windbridge Institute, LLC

Jackson, Laura Lynne (2016) *The Light Between Us: Stories from Heaven. Lessons for the Living.* New York: Spiegel & Grau.

Jackson, Laura Lynne (2020) *Signs: The Secret Language of the Universe.* New York: Random House.

Russo, Kim (2017) *The Happy Medium: Life Lessons from the Other Side.* New York: HarperOne.

Russo, Kim (2020) *Your Soul Purpose: Learn How to Access the Light Within.* New York: HarperOne.

## PSI RESEARCH/PARAPSYCHOLOGY

Cheung, Theresa, Julia Mossbridge, Loyd Auerbach, and Dean Radin (2018) *The Premonition Code: The Science of Precognition, How Sensing the Future Can Change Your Life*. London: Watkins Publishing.

Radin, Dean (2018) *Real Magic: Ancient Wisdom, Modern Science, and a Guide to the Secret Power of the Universe*. New York: Harmony Books.

Radin, Dean (2013) *Supernormal: Science, Yoga, and the Evidence for Extraordinary Psychic Abilities*. La Jolla, Calif.: Deepak Chopra Books.

## SURVIVAL/REINCARNATION RESEARCH

Fontana, David (2005) *Is There An Afterlife?: A Comprehensive Overview of the Evidence*. Winchester, UK: Iff Books.

Holden, Janice Miner, Bruce Greyson, and Debbie James (Eds.) (2009) *The Handbook of Near-Death Experiences: Thirty Years of Investigation*. Westport, Conn.: Praeger.

Horn, Stacy (2010) *Unbelievable: Investigations into Ghosts, Poltergeists, Telepathy, and Other Unseen Phenomena, from the Duke Parapsychology Laboratory*. New York: Ecco.

Kean, Leslie (2017) *Surviving Death: A Journalist Investigates Evidence for an Afterlife*. New York: Crown Archetype.

Rock, Adam J. (2014) *The Survival Hypothesis: Essays on Mediumship*. Jefferson, N.C.: McFarland & Co.

Tucker, Jim B., and Ian Stevenson (2008) *Life Before Life: Children's Memories of Previous Lives*. New York: St. Martin's Publishing Group.

# Bibliography

Abraham, Henry David (1983) "Visual Phenomenology of the LSD Flashback." *Archives of General Psychiatry* 40 (8): 884–89.

Aglioti, S., N. Smania, M. Manfredi, and G. Berlucchi (1996) "Disownership of Left Hand and Objects Related to It in a Patient with Right Brain Damage." *NeuroReport* 8 (1): 293–96.

Alderson-Day, B. (2016) "The Silent Companions." *Psychologist* 29 (4): 272–75.

Anchisi, Davide, and Marco Zanon (2015) "A Bayesian Perspective on Sensory and Cognitive Integration in Pain Perception and Placebo Analgesia." Edited by Jean Daunizeau. *PLOS One* 10 (2): e0117270.

Arzy, S., and R. Schurr (2016) "'God Has Sent Me to You': Right Temporal Epilepsy, Left Prefrontal Psychosis." *Epilepsy & Behavior* 60: 7–10.

Atasoy, Selen, Gustavo Deco, Morten L. Kringelbach, and Joel Pearson (2018) "Harmonic Brain Modes: A Unifying Framework for Linking Space and Time in Brain Dynamics." *Neuroscientist*. SAGE Publications Inc.

Atasoy, Selen, Isaac Donnelly, and Joel Pearson (2016) "Human Brain Networks Function in Connectome-Specific Harmonic Waves." *Nature Communications* 7 (January).

Atasoy, Selen, Leor Roseman, Mendel Kaelen, Morten L. Kringelbach, Gustavo Deco, and Robin L. Carhart-Harris (2017) "Connectome-Harmonic Decomposition of Human Brain Activity Reveals Dynamical Repertoire Re-Organization under LSD." *Scientific Reports* 7 (1).

Atlas, Lauren Y., and Tor D. Wager (2012) "How Expectations Shape Pain." *Neuroscience Letters* 520 (2): 140–48.

Aviezer, Hillel, Shlomo Bentin, Veronica Dudarev, and Ran R. Hassin (2011)

"The Automaticity of Emotional Face-Context Integration." *Emotion* 11 (6): 1406–14.

Balcetis, Emily, and David Dunning (2006) "See What You Want to See: Motivational Influences on Visual Perception." *Journal of Personality and Social Psychology* 91 (4): 612–25.

Balcetis, Emily, David Dunning, and Yael Granot (2012) "Subjective Value Determines Initial Dominance in Binocular Rivalry." *Journal of Experimental Social Psychology* 48 (1): 122–29.

Balestrini, S., S. Francione, R. Mai, L. Castana, G. Casaceli, Daniela Marino, Leandro Provinciali, Francesco Cardinale, and Laura Tassi (2015) "Multimodal Responses Induced by Cortical Stimulation of the Parietal Lobe: A Stereo-Electroencephalography Study." *Brain* 138 (9): 2596–2607.

Ballard, Jamie (2019, October 21) "Many Americans Believe Ghosts and Demons Exist." YouGov America.

Baptista, Johann, Max Derakhshani, and Patrizio Tressoldi (2015) "Explicit Anomalous Cognition: A Review of the Best Evidence in Ganzfeld, Forced-Choice, Remote Viewing and Dream Studies." *Parapsychology: A Handbook for the 21st Century*. Edited by Etzel Cardeña, John Palmer, and David Marcusson-Clavertz. Jefferson, N.C.: McFarland & Company, Inc. 192–214.

Barreiro, Julio T. (2011) "Environmental Effects Controlled." *Nature Physics* 7 (12): 927–28.

Barušs, Imants, and Julia Mossbridge (2017) *Transcendent Mind: Rethinking the Science of Consciousness*. Washington, D.C.: American Psychological Association.

Battelli, L., A. Pascual-Leone, and P. Cavanagh (2007) "The 'When' Pathway of the Right Parietal Lobe." *Trends in Cognitive Sciences* 11 (5): 204–10.

Bear, David M., and Paul Fedio (1977) "Quantitative Analysis of Interictal Behavior in Temporal Lobe Epilepsy." *Archives of Neurology* 34 (8): 454–67.

Behrendt, R. P. (2013) "Hippocampus and Consciousness." *Reviews in the Neurosciences* 24 (3): 239–66.

Beischel, J., C. Mosher, and M. Boccuzzi (2017) "Quantitative and Qualitative Analyses of Mediumistic and Psychic Experiences." *Threshold: Journal of Interdisciplinary Consciousness Studies* 1 (2).

Bell, John S. (1964) "On the Einstein Podolsky Rosen Paradox." *Physics Physique Fizika* 1 (3): 195.

Bem, Daryl J. (2011) "Feeling the Future: Experimental Evidence for Anomalous

Retroactive Influences on Cognition and Affect." *Journal of Personality and Social Psychology* 100 (3): 407–25.

Bem, Daryl J., and Charles Honorton (1994) "Does Psi Exist? Replicable Evidence for an Anomalous Process of Information Transfer." *Psychological Bulletin* 115 (1).

Bem, Daryl J., Patrizio Tressoldi, Thomas Rabeyron, and Michael Duggan (2016) "Feeling the Future: A Meta-Analysis of 90 Experiments on the Anomalous Anticipation of Random Future Events." *F1000Research* (4).

Berkovich-Ohana, A., M. Harel, A. Hahamy, A. Arieli, and R. Malach (2016) "Data for Default Network Reduced Functional Connectivity in Meditators, Negatively Correlated with Meditation Expertise." *Data in Brief* 8: 910–14.

Berlucchi, G., and S. Aglioti (1997) "The Body in the Brain: Neural Bases of Corporeal Awareness." *Trends in Neurosciences* 20 (12): 560–64.

Blanke, O., T. Landis, L. Spinelli, and M. Seeck (2004) "Out-of-Body Experience and Autoscopy of Neurological Origin." *Brain* 127 (2): 243–58.

Blanke, Olaf, Christine Mohr, Christoph M. Michel, Alvaro Pascual-Leone, Peter Brugger, Margitta Seeck, Theodor Landis, and Gregor Thut (2005) "Linking Out-of-Body Experience and Self Processing to Mental Own-Body Imagery at the Temporoparietal Junction." *Journal of Neuroscience* 25 (3): 550–57.

Blanke, O., S. Ortigue, T. Landis, and M. Seeck (2002) "Stimulating Illusory Own-Body Perceptions." *Nature* 419 (6904): 269–70.

Blewett, D. B., and N. Chwelos (1959) "Handbook for the Therapeutic Use of LSD-25: Individual and Group Procedures." Multidisciplinary Association for Psychedelic Studies.

Blom, Jan Dirk (2010) *A Dictionary of Hallucinations*. New York: Springer.

Booth, Mark (2008) *The Secret History of the World*. New York: The Overlook Press.

Bösch, Holger, Fiona Steinkamp, and Emil Boller (2006) "Examining Psychokinesis: The Interaction of Human Intention With Random Number Generators—A Meta-Analysis." *Psychological Bulletin* 132 (4): 497.

Brugger, P. (2006) "From Phantom Limb to Phantom Body: Varieties of Extracorporeal Awareness." *Human Body Perception from the Inside Out*. Edited by G. Knoblich, I. M. Thornton, M. Grosjean, and M. Shiffrar. Oxford: Oxford University Press: 171–209.

Buckner, Randy L., Jessica R. Andrews-Hanna, and Daniel L. Schacter (2008)

"The Brain's Default Network Anatomy, Function, and Relevance to Disease." *Annals of the New York Academy of Sciences* 1124: 1–38.

Bueti, Domenica, and Vincent Walsh (2009) "The Parietal Cortex and the Representation of Time, Space, Number and Other Magnitudes." *Philosophical Transactions of the Royal Society B: Biological Sciences* 364 (1525): 1831–40.

Cardeña, Etzel (2014) "A Call for an Open, Informed Study of All Aspects of Consciousness." *Frontiers in Human Neuroscience* 8 (January): 17.

Cardeña, Etzel (2018) "The Experimental Evidence for Parapsychological Phenomena: A Review." *American Psychologist* 73 (5): 663–77.

Cardeña, Etzel, John Palmer, and David Marcusson-Clavertz, eds. (2015) *Parapsychology: A Handbook for the 21st Century.* Jefferson, N.C.: McFarland & Company, Inc.

Carhart-Harris, Robin L, David Erritzoe, Tim Williams, James M. Stone, Laurence J. Reed, Alessandro Colasanti, Robin J. Tyacke, et al. (2012) "Neural Correlates of the Psychedelic State as Determined by fMRI Studies with Psilocybin." *National Academy of Sciences* 109 (6): 2138–43.

Carhart-Harris, R., R. Leech, and E. Tagliazucchi (2014) "How Do Hallucinogens Work on the Brain?" *Journal of Psychophysiology* 71 (1): 2–8.

Carney, Dana R., Amy J. C. Cuddy, and Andy J. Yap (2010) "Power Posing." *Psychological Science* 21 (10): 1363–68.

Cavanna, A. E., and M. R. Trimble (2006) "The Precuneus: A Review of Its Functional Anatomy and Behavioural Correlates." *Brain* 129 (3): 564–83.

Center for Humane Technology (2021, February 11) "A Renegade Solution to Extractive Economics." Your Undivided Attention.

Chalmers, David J. (1995) *The Conscious Mind. In Search of a Fundamental Theory.* Oxford: Oxford University Press.

Chalmers, David J. (2003) "Consciousness and Its Place in Nature." *The Blackwell Guide to Philosophy of Mind.* Hoboken, NJ: Blackwell Publishing Ltd.: 102–42.

Cheyne, J. A. (2001) "The Ominous Numinous: Sensed Presence and 'Other' Hallucinations." *Journal of Consciousness Studies* 8 (5–6): 133–50.

Cleary, T. (1993) *The Flower Ornament Scripture: A Translation of the Avatamsaka Sutra.* Boulder, Colo.: Shambhala Publications.

Cohen, Jacob. (1992) "A Power Primer." *Psychological Bulletin* 112 (1): 155–59.

Cohen, Jacob. (2013) *Statistical Power Analysis for the Behavioral Sciences. Statistical Power Analysis for the Behavioral Sciences.* Cambridge: Academic Press.

Cole, Shana, Emily Balcetis, and David Dunning (2013) "Affective Signals of Threat Increase Perceived Proximity." *Psychological Science* 24 (1): 34–40.

Colloca, Luana (2018) "Preface: The Fascinating Mechanisms and Implications of the Placebo Effect." *International Review of Neurobiology*. Cambridge: Academic Press.

Cook, C. M., and M. A. Persinger (1997) "Experimental Induction of the 'Sensed Presence' in Normal Subjects and an Exceptional Subject." *Perceptual and Motor Skills* 85 (2): 683–93.

Cooper, Anderson (2019, August 16) "Interview of Stephen Colbert." *Anderson Cooper 360°*.

Cranston, S., and C. Williams (1984) *Reincarnation: A New Horizon In Science, Religion And Society*. New York: Julian Press.

Crescentini, C., M. Di Bucchianico, F. Fabbro, and C. Urgesi (2015) "Excitatory Stimulation of the Right Inferior Parietal Cortex Lessens Implicit Religiousness/Spirituality." *Neuropsychologia* 70: 71–79.

Crescentini, C., C. Urgesi, F. Campanella, Roberto Eleopra, and Franco Fabbro (2014) "Effects of an 8-Week Meditation Program on the Implicit and Explicit Attitudes toward Religious/Spiritual Self-Representations." *Consciousness and Cognition* 30: 266–80.

Crick, Francis, and Christof Koch (2003) "A Framework for Consciousness." *Nature Neuroscience*. Nature Publishing Group.

Daltrozzo, Jerome, Boris Kotchoubey, Fatma Gueler, and Ahmed A. Karim (2016) "Effects of Transcranial Magnetic Stimulation on Body Perception: No Evidence for Specificity of the Right Temporo-Parietal Junction." *Brain Topography* 29 (5): 704–15.

Damisch, Lysann, Barbara Stoberock, and Thomas Mussweiler (2010) "Keep Your Fingers Crossed! How Superstition Improves Performance." *Psychological Science* 21 (7): 1014–20.

Davis, Alan K., Frederick S. Barrett, and Roland R. Griffiths (2020) "Psychological Flexibility Mediates the Relations between Acute Psychedelic Effects and Subjective Decreases in Depression and Anxiety." *Journal of Contextual Behavioral Science* 15: 39–45.

Davis, Alan K., John M. Clifton, Eric G. Weaver, Ethan S. Hurwitz, Matthew W. Johnson, and Roland R. Griffiths (2020) "Survey of Entity Encounter Experiences Occasioned by Inhaled N,N-Dimethyltryptamine: Phenomenology, Interpretation, and Enduring Effects." *Journal of Psychopharmacology* 34 (9): 1008–20.

Davisson, C., and L. H. Germer (1927) "The Scattering of Electrons by a Single Crystal of Nickel." *Nature* 119 (2998): 558–60.

Decety, J., and C. Lamm (2007) "The Role of the Right Temporoparietal Junction in Social Interaction: How Low-Level Computational Processes Contribute to Meta-Cognition." *The Neuroscientist* 13 (6): 580–93.

Denny, Bryan T., Hedy Kober, Tor D. Wager, and Kevin N. Ochsner (2012) "A Meta-Analysis of Functional Neuroimaging Studies of Self- and Other Judgments Reveals a Spatial Gradient for Mentalizing in Medial Prefrontal Cortex." *Journal of Cognitive Neuroscience* 24 (8): 1742–52.

De Ridder, Dirk, Koen Van Laere, Patrick Dupont, Tomas Menovsky, and Paul Van de Heyning (2007) "Visualizing Out-of-Body Experience in the Brain." *New England Journal of Medicine* 357 (18): 1829–33.

Desmedt, John E., and Claude Tomberg (1994) "Transient Phase-Locking of 40 Hz Electrical Oscillations in Prefrontal and Parietal Human Cortex Reflects the Process of Conscious Somatic Perception." *Neuroscience Letters* 168 (1–2): 126–29.

Devereux, Paul (1997) *The Long Trip: A Prehistory of Psychedelia*. New York: Penguin Arkana.

Diekhof, Esther K., Hanne E. Kipshagen, Peter Falkai, Peter Dechent, Jürgen Baudewig, and Oliver Gruber (2011) "The Power of Imagination: How Anticipatory Mental Imagery Alters Perceptual Processing of Fearful Facial Expressions." *NeuroImage* 54 (2): 1703–14.

Dijksterhuis, Ap, and Henk Aarts (2003) "On Wildebeests and Humans: The Preferential Detection of Negative Stimuli." *Psychological Science* 14 (1): 14–8.

Dijksterhuis, Ap, Maarten W. Bos, Loran F. Nordgren, and Rick B. Van Baaren (2006) "On Making the Right Choice: The Deliberation-without-Attention Effect." *Science* 311 (5763): 1005–7.

Doesburg, Sam M., Jessica J. Green, John J. McDonald, and Lawrence M. Ward (2009) "Rhythms of Consciousness: Binocular Rivalry Reveals Large-Scale Oscillatory Network Dynamics Mediating Visual Perception." *PLOS One* 4 (7): 6142.

Dossey, Larry (1999) *Reinventing Medicine: Beyond Mind-Body to a New Era of Healing*. San Francisco: Harper Collins.

Ducasse, C. J. (1960) " How the Case of The Search for Bridey Murphy Stands Today." *The Journal of the American Society for Psychical Research* 54 (January): 3–22.

Duggan, Michael, and Patrizio Tressoldi (2018) "Predictive Physiological Anticipatory Activity Preceding Seemingly Unpredictable Stimuli: An Update of Mossbridge et al's Meta-Analysis." *F1000Research* (7): 407.

Dunne, Brenda J., and Robert G. Jahn (2003) "Information and Uncertainty in Remote Perception Research." *Journal of Scientific Exploration* 17 (2): 207–41.

Dunning, Jonathan P., Muhammad A. Parvaz, Greg Hajcak, Thomas Maloney, Nelly Alia-Klein, Patricia A. Woicik, Frank Telang, Gene-Jack Wang, Nora D. Volkow, and Rita Z. Goldstein (2011) "Motivated Attention to Cocaine and Emotional Cues in Abstinent and Current Cocaine Users: an ERP Study." *European Journal of Neuroscience* 33 (9): 1716–23.

Eagleman, David (2011) *Incognito: The Secret Lives of the Brain*. New York: Pantheon.

Eastwood, John D., Daniel Smilek, and Philip M. Merikle (2001) "Differential Attentional Guidance by Unattended Faces Expressing Positive and Negative Emotion." *Perception and Psychophysics* 63 (6): 1004–13.

Eimer, Martin, and Amanda Holmes (2002) "An ERP Study on the Time Course of Emotional Face Processing." *NeuroReport* 13 (4): 427–31.

Engel, Andreas K., and Wolf Singer (2001) "Temporal Binding and the Neural Correlates of Sensory Awareness." *Trends in Cognitive Sciences* 5 (1): 16–25.

Engel, G. S., T. R. Calhoun, E. L. Read, T. K. Ahn, T. Mančal, Y. C. Cheng, R. E. Blankenship, and G. R. Fleming (2007) "Evidence for Wavelike Energy Transfer through Quantum Coherence in Photosynthetic Systems." *Nature* 446 (7137): 782–86.

Fallon, Nicholas, Carl Roberts, and Andrej Stancak (2020) "Shared and Distinct Functional Networks for Empathy and Pain Processing: A Systematic Review and Meta-Analysis of fMRI Studies." *Social Cognitive and Affective Neuroscience* 15 (7): 709–23.

Feynman, Richard (1967) *The Character of Physical Law*. Cambridge, Mass.: MIT Press.

Fiore, Edith (1978) *You Have Been Here before: A Psychologist Looks at Past Lives*. New York: Coward, McCann & Geoghegan.

Fox, K. C. R., M. L. Dixon, S. Nijeboer, M. Girn, J. L. Floman, M. Lifshitz, M. Ellamil, P. Sedlmeier, and K. Christoff (2016) "Functional Neuroanatomy of Meditation: A Review and Meta-Analysis of 78 Functional Neuroimaging Investigations." *Neuroscience & Biobehavioral Reviews* 65: 208–28.

Fox, Michael D., Abraham Z. Snyder, Justin L. Vincent, Maurizio Corbetta,

David C. Van Essen, and Marcus E. Raichle (2005) "The Human Brain Is Intrinsically Organized into Dynamic, Anticorrelated Functional Networks." *Proceedings of the National Academy of Sciences* 102 (27): 9673–78.

Friedrich, Alena, Barbara Flunger, Benjamin Nagengast, Kathrin Jonkmann, and Ulrich Trautwein (2015) "Pygmalion Effects in the Classroom: Teacher Expectancy Effects on Students' Math Achievement." *Contemporary Educational Psychology* 41 (April): 1–12.

Gaillard, Raphaël, Stanislas Dehaene, Claude Adam, Stéphane Clémenceau, Dominique Hasboun, Michel Baulac, Laurent Cohen, and Lionel Naccache (2009) "Converging Intracranial Markers of Conscious Access." Edited by Leslie Ungerleider. *PLOS Biology* 7 (3): e1000061.

Gazzaniga, Michael S. (2005) "Forty-Five Years of Split-Brain Research and Still Going Strong." *Nature Reviews Neuroscience* 6: 653–659.

Gazzaniga, Michael S. (1970) *Neuroscience Series*. Vol. 2: *The Bisected Brain*. New York: Appleton-Century-Crofts.

Geschwind, Norman (1983) "Interictal Behavioral Changes in Epilepsy." *Epilepsia* 24: S23–30.

Goff, Philip (2017) *Consciousness and Fundamental Reality*. Oxford: Oxford University Press.

Goff, Philip (2018, February 8) "Cosmopsychism Explains Why the Universe Is Fine-Tuned for Life." Aeon.

Goleman, Daniel, and Richard J. Davidson (2017) *Altered Traits: Science Reveals How Meditation Changes Your Mind, Brain, and Body*. New York: Avery Publishing.

Good, Thomas L., Natasha Sterzinger, and Alyson Lavigne (2018) "Expectation Effects: Pygmalion and the Initial 20 Years of Research1." *Educational Research and Evaluation* 24 (3–5): 99–123.

Griffiths, R. R., W. A. Richards, U. McCann, and R. Jesse (2006) "Psilocybin Can Occasion Mystical-Type Experiences Having Substantial and Sustained Personal Meaning and Spiritual Significance." *Psychopharmacology* 187 (3): 268–83.

Grof, S. (1988) *The Adventure of Self-Discovery: Dimensions of Consciousness and New Perspectives in Psychotherapy and Inner Exploration*. Albany: State University of New York Press.

Grof, S. (2001) *LSD Psychotherapy*. 3rd ed. Sarasota, Fla.: Multidisciplinary Association for Psychedelic Studies.

Grof, S. (1975) "Varieties of Transpersonal Experiences: Observations from LSD

Psychotherapy." *Psychiatry and Mysticism.* Edited by SR Dean. Chicago: Nelson-Hall: 311–45.

Gronau, Quentin F., Sara Van Erp, Daniel W. Heck, Joseph Cesario, Kai J. Jonas, and Eric Jan Wagenmakers (2017) "A Bayesian Model-Averaged Meta-Analysis of the Power Pose Effect with Informed and Default Priors: The Case of Felt Power." *Comprehensive Results in Social Psychology* 2 (1): 123–38.

Haidich, A. B. (2010) "Meta-Analysis in Medical Research." *Hippokratia* 14 (Suppl 1): 29-undefined.

Handler, Chelsea (2019) *Life Will Be the Death of Me.* New York: The Dial Press.

Handler, Chelsea (2019, September 25) "People on the Other Side with Laura Lynne Jackson." *Life Will Be the Death of Me.* iHeart.

Harman, Willis W. (1963) "Some Aspects of the Psychedelic-Drug Controversy." *Journal of Humanistic Psychology* 3 (2): 93–107.

Head, Joseph, and Sylvia L. Cranston (1977) *Reincarnation: The Phoenix Fire Mystery: An East-West Dialogue on Death and Rebirth from the Worlds of Religion, Science, Psychology, Philosophy, Art, and and Literature, and from Great Thinkers of the Past and Present.* New York: Julian Press.

Herbet, Guillaume, Gilles Lafargue, Nicolas Menjot de Champfleur, Sylvie Moritz-Gasser, Emmanuelle Le Bars, François Bonnetblanc, and Hugues Duffau (2014) "Disrupting Posterior Cingulate Connectivity Disconnects Consciousness from the External Environment." *Neuropsychologia* 56: 239–44.

Hermle, Leo, Matthias Fünfgeld, Godehard Oepen, Hanno Botsch, Dieter Borchardt, Euphrosyne Gouzoulis, Rose A. Fehrenbach, and Manfred Spitzer (1992) "Mescaline-Induced Psychopathological, Neuropsychological, and Neurometabolic Effects in Normal Subjects: Experimental Psychosis as a Tool for Psychiatric Research." *Biological Psychiatry* 32 (11): 976–91.

Hoffman, Donald (2019) *The Case Against Reality: Why Evolution Hid the Truth from Our Eyes.* New York: W. W. Norton & Company.

Holt, Nicola J., Deborah L. Delanoy, and Chris A. Roe (2004) "Creativity, Subjective Paranormal Experiences and Altered States of Consciousness." *The Parapsychological Association, 47th Annual Convention:* 433–36.

Holzinger, Rudolf (1964) "LSD-25, A Tool in Psychotherapy." *The Journal of General Psychology* 71 (1): 9–20.

Honorton, C., and D. C. Ferrari (1989) "'Future Telling': A Meta-Analysis of Forced-Choice Precognition Experiments, 1935–1987." *Journal of Parapsychology* 53: 281–308.

Humphreys, G. F., and M. A. Lambon Ralph (2015) "Fusion and Fission of Cognitive Functions in the Human Parietal Cortex." *Cerebral Cortex* 25 (10): 3547–60.

Huxley, Aldous (1954). *The Doors of Perception.* London. Chatto & Windus.

Hyman, Ray (1995) "Evaluation of Program on Anomalous Mental Phenomena." *Journal of Scientific Exploration* 10 (1): 31–58.

Hyman, Ray (1985) "The Ganzfeld Psi Experiment: A Critical Appraisal." *The Journal of Parapsychology* 49 (1): 3-undefined.

Ionta, Silvio, Roger Gassert, and Olaf Blanke (2011) "Multi-Sensory and Sensorimotor Foundation of Bodily Self-Consciousness: an Interdisciplinary Approach." *Frontiers in Psychology* 2 (December): 383.

Ionta, S., L. Heydrich, B. Lenggenhager, M. Mouthon, Eleonora Fornari, Dominique Chapuis, Roger Gassert, and Olaf Blanke (2011) "Multisensory Mechanisms in Temporo-Parietal Cortex Support Self-Location and First-Person Perspective." *Neuron* 70 (2): 363–72.

Jacobsen, Annie (2017) *Phenomena: The Secret History of the U.S. Government's Investigations into Extrasensory Perception and Psychokinesis.* New York: Little, Brown and Company.

Johanson, Mika, Olli Vaurio, Jari Tiihonen, and Markku Lähteenvuo (2020) "A Systematic Literature Review of Neuroimaging of Psychopathic Traits." *Frontiers in Psychiatry* 10 (February): 1027.

Josipovic, Zoran (2010) "Duality and Nonduality in Meditation Research." *Consciousness and Cognition* 19 (4): 1119–21.

Josipovic, Zoran, Ilan Dinstein, Jochen Weber, and David J. Heeger (2012) "Influence of Meditation on Anti-Correlated Networks in the Brain." *Frontiers in Human Neuroscience* 5 (January): 1–11.

Kahneman, Daniel (2011) *Thinking, Fast and Slow.* New York: Macmillan.

Kahneman, Daniel., Dan Lovallo, and Olivier Sibony (2011) "Before You Make That Big Decision." *Harvard Business Review* 89 (6): 50–60.

Kaptchuk, Ted J., Elizabeth Friedlander, John M. Kelley, M. Norma Sanchez, Efi Kokkotou, Joyce P. Singer, Magda Kowalczykowski, Franklin G. Miller, Irving Kirsch, and Anthony J. Lembo (2010) "Placebos without Deception: A Randomized Controlled Trial in Irritable Bowel Syndrome." Edited by Isabelle Boutron. *PLOS One* 5 (12): e15591.

Kastrup, Bernardo (2018) "The Universe in Consciousness." *Journal of Consciousness Studies* (25): 5–6.

Kastrup, Bernardo (2014) *Why Materialism Is Baloney: How True Skeptics Know There Is No Death and Fathom Answers to Life, the Universe, and Everything.* Hampshire, U.K.: John Hunt Publishing.

Kastrup, Bernardo, Adam Crabtree, and Edward F. Kelly (2018, June 18) "Could Multiple Personality Disorder Explain Life, the Universe and Everything?" *Scientific American Blog Network.* (June) *Scientific American.*

Kelley, W. M., C. N. Macrae, C. L. Wyland, S. Caglar, S. Inati, and T. F. Heatherton (2002) "Finding the Self? An Event-Related fMRI Study." *Journal of Cognitive Neuroscience* 14: 785–94.

Kelly, Edward F., Adam Crabtree, and Paul Marshall (Eds.) (2015) *Beyond Physicalism: Toward Reconciliation of Science and Spirituality.* Lanham, Md.: Rowman & Littlefield.

Kelly, Edward F., Emily Williams Kelly, Adam Crabtree, Alan Gauld, and Michael Grosso, eds. (2007) *Irreducible Mind: Toward a Psychology for the 21st Century.* Lanham, Md.: Rowman & Littlefield.

Kelly, Edward F., and Paul Marshall, eds. (2021) *Consciousness Unbound: Liberating Mind from the Tyranny of Materialism.* Lanham, Md.: Rowman & Littlefield.

Kelly, Emily Williams (2007) "Unusual Experiences Near Death and Related Phenomena." *Irreducible Mind: Toward a Psychology for the 21st Century.* Edited by E. F. Kelly, E. W. Kelly, A. Crabtree, A. Gauld, and M. Grosso. Lanham, Md.: Rowman & Littlefield.

Keppler, Joachim (2012) "A Conceptual Framework for Consciousness Based on a Deep Understanding of Matter." *Philosophy Study* 2 (10): 689–703.

Keppler, Joachim, and Itay Shani (2020) "Cosmopsychism and Consciousness Research: A Fresh View on the Causal Mechanisms Underlying Phenomenal States." *Frontiers in Psychology* 11 (March) 371.

Kim, Yoon Ho, Rong Yu, Sergei P. Kulik, and Marlan O. Scully (2000) "Delayed 'Choice' Quantum Eraser." *Physical Review Letters* 84 (1): 1–5.

King, Lester S. (1975) "Cases of the Reincarnation Type, Vol. 1: Ten Cases in India." *JAMA: The Journal of the American Medical Association* 234 (9): 978.

Koch, Christof (2012) *Consciousness: Confessions of a Romantic Reductionist.* Cambridge, Mass.: MIT Press.

Kolbaba, Scott J. (2016) *Physicians' Untold Stories: Miraculous Experiences*

*Doctors Are Hesitant to Share with Their Patients, or ANYONE!* Scotts Valley, Calif.: Createspace Independent Publishing Platform.

Kometer, Michael, Thomas Pokorny, Erich Seifritz, and Franz X. Volleinweider (2015) "Psilocybin-Induced Spiritual Experiences and Insightfulness Are Associated with Synchronization of Neuronal Oscillations." *Psychopharmacology* 232 (19): 3663–76.

Kometer, Michael, André Schmidt, Lutz Jäncke, and Franz X. Vollenweider (2013) "Activation of Serotonin 2A Receptors Underlies the Psilocybin-Induced Effects on α Oscillations, N170 Visual-Evoked Potentials, and Visual Hallucinations." *Journal of Neuroscience* 33 (25): 10544–51.

Kominis, Iannis K. (2015) "The Radical-Pair Mechanism as a Paradigm for the Emerging Science of Quantum Biology." *Modern Physics Letters B* 29 (1): 1530013.

Kripal, Jeffrey J. (2019) *The Flip: Epiphanies of Mind and the Future of Knowledge.* New York: Bellevue Literary Press.

Kubit, Benjamin, and Anthony Ian Jack (2013) "Rethinking the Role of the RTPJ in Attention and Social Cognition in Light of the Opposing Domains Hypothesis: Findings from an ALE-Based Meta-Analysis and Resting-State Functional Connectivity." *Frontiers in Human Neuroscience* 7 (June): 323.

Kurzweil, Ray (2013) *How to Create a Mind: The Secret of Human Thought Revealed.* New York: Penguin Books.

Lamont, Ruth A., Hannah J. Swift, and Dominic Abrams (2015) "A Review and Meta-Analysis of Age-Based Stereotype Threat: Negative Stereotypes, Not Facts, Do the Damage." *Psychology and Aging* 30 (1): 180–93.

Leslie, Paul J. (2019) *Shadows in the Session: The Presence of the Anomalous in Psychotherapy.* Path Notes Press.

Leucht, Stefan, Bartosz Helfer, Gerald Gartlehner, and John M. Davis (2015) "How Effective Are Common Medications: A Perspective Based on Meta-Analyses of Major Drugs." *BMC Medicine* 13 (October): 253.

Lick, D. J., A. L. Alter, and J. B. Freeman (2018) "Superior Pattern Detectors Efficiently Learn, Activate, Apply, and Update Social Stereotypes." *Journal of Experimental Psychology* 147 (2): 209–27.

Lommel, P. Van, R. Van Wees, V. Meyers, and I. Elfferich (2001) "Near-Death Experience in Survivors of Cardiac Arrest: A Prospective Study in the Netherlands." *The Lancet* 358 (9298): 2039–45.

Long, Jeffrey, and Jody Long (1999) "Near Death Experience (NDE) Overview." Near-Death Experience Research Foundation.

Luhrmann, Tanya M. (2012) *When God Talks Back: Understanding the American Evangelical Relationship with God.* New York: Knopf Doubleday Publishing Group.

Luke, David P. (2012) "Psychoactive Substances and Paranormal Phenomena: A Comprehensive Review." *International Journal of Transpersonal Studies* 31 (1): 97–156.

Luke, David P., and Marios Kittenis (2005) "A Preliminary Survey of Paranormal Experiences with Psychoactive Drugs." *The Journal of Parapsychology* 69 (2): 305.

Luppi, Andrea I., Jakub Vohryzek, Morten L. Kringelbach, Pedro A. M. Mediano, M. M. Craig, Ram Adapa, R. L. Carhart-Harris, et al. (2020) "Connectome Harmonic Decomposition of Human Brain Dynamics Reveals a Landscape of Consciousness." *bioRxiv* (August 10): 244459.

Lutkajtis, Anna (2021) "Entity Encounters and the Therapeutic Effect of the Psychedelic Mystical Experience." *Journal of Psychedelic Studies* 4 (3): 171–78.

Lutz, A., H. A. Slagter, J. D. Dunne, and R. J. Davidson (2008) "Attention Regulation and Monitoring in Meditation." *Trends in Cognitive Sciences* 12 (4): 163–69.

Maner, Jon K., Matthew T. Gailliot, D. Aaron Rouby, and Saul L. Miller (2007) "Can't Take My Eyes off You: Attentional Adhesion to Mates and Rivals." *Journal of Personality and Social Psychology* 93 (3): 389–401.

Manning, A. G., R. I. Khakimov, R. G. Dall, and A. G. Truscott (2015) "Wheeler's Delayed-Choice Gedanken Experiment with a Single Atom." *Nature Physics* 11 (7): 539–542.

Mathews, Freya (2011) "Panpsychism as Paradigm." *The Mental as Fundamental: New Perspectives on Panpsychism.* Edited by M. Blamauer. Heusenstamm, Ger.: Ontos Verlag: 141–56.

May, Edwin C., Jessica M. Utts, Virginia V. Trask, Wanda W. Luke, Thand J. Frivold, and Beverley S. Humphrey (1989) "Review of the Psychoenergetic Research Conducted at SRI International (1973–1988)." *Menlo Park* 33: 1–25.

McConnell, R. A., and T. K. Clarke (1991) "National Academy of Sciences' Opinion on Parapsychology." *Journal of the American Society for Psychical Research* 85 (4): 333–65.

McKenna, Terence (1999) *Food of the Gods: The Search for the Original Tree of Knowledge: a Radical History of Plants, Drugs and Human Evolution.* New York: Random House.

Melloni, Lucia, Carlos Molina, Marcela Pena, David Torres, Wolf Singer, and Eugenio Rodriguez (2007) "Synchronization of Neural Activity across Cortical Areas Correlates with Conscious Perception." *Journal of Neuroscience* 27 (11): 2858–65.

Mertens, Gaëtan, and Iris M. Engelhard (2020) "A Systematic Review and Meta-Analysis of the Evidence for Unaware Fear Conditioning." *Neuroscience and Biobehavioral Reviews* 108: 254–268.

Mills, A., E. Haraldsson, and H. J. Keil (1994) "Replication Studies of Cases Suggestive of Reincarnation by Three Independent Investigators." *Journal of the American Society for Psychical Research* 88 (3): 207–19.

Mills, Antonia and Jim B. Tucker (2015) "Reincarnation: Field Studies and Theoretical Issues Today." *Parapsychology: A Handbook for the 21st Century.* Edited by Etzel Cardeña, John Palmer, and David Marcusson-Clavertz. Jefferson, N.C.: McFarland & Company, Inc., Publishers: 314–326.

Milton, J. (1997) "Meta-Analysis of Free-Response ESP Studies without Altered States of Consciousness." *The Journal of Parapsychology* 61 (4): 279.

Milton, Julie, and Richard Wiseman (1999) "Does Psi Exist? Lack of Replication of an Anomalous Process of Information Transfer." *Psychological Bulletin* 125 (4): 387.

Moore, David W. (2005, June 16) "Three in Four Americans Believe in Paranormal." Gallup Poll News Service.

Mossbridge, Julia (2016) "Designing Transcendence Technology." *Psychology's New Design Science and the Reflective Practitioner.* Edited by Susan Imholz, and Judy Sachter. River Bend, N.C.: LibraLab Press.

Mossbridge, Julia, Patrizio Tressoldi, and Jessica Utts (2012) "Predictive Physiological Anticipation Preceding Seemingly Unpredictable Stimuli: A Meta-Analysis." *Frontiers in Psychology* 3 (October): 390.

Mossbridge, Julia A., Patrizio Tressoldi, Jessica Utts, John A. Ives, Dean Radin, and Wayne B. Jonas (2014) "Predicting the Unpredictable: Critical Analysis and Practical Implications of Predictive Anticipatory Activity." *Frontiers in Human Neuroscience* 8: 146.

Muthukumaraswamy, Suresh D., Robin L. Carhart-Harris, Rosalyn J. Moran, Matthew J. Brookes, Tim M. Williams, David Errtizoe, Ben Sessa, et al. (2013) "Broadband Cortical Desynchronization Underlies the Human Psychedelic State." *Journal of Neuroscience* 33 (38): 15171–83.

Nagasawa, Yujin, and K. Wager (2017) "Panpsychism and Priority Cosmopsychism." *Panpsychism: Contemporary Perspectives.* Edited by

G. Brüntrup and L. Jaskolla. Oxford: Oxford University Press: 113–29.

Nahm, Michael, Bruce Greyson, Emily Williams Kelly, and Erlendur Haraldsson (2012) "Terminal Lucidity: A Review and a Case Collection." *Archives of Gerontology and Geriatrics* 55 (1): 138–42.

Nash, Jonathan D., and Andrew Newberg (2013) "Toward a Unifying Taxonomy and Definition for Meditation." *Frontiers in Psychology* 4 (November): 806.

National Alliance on Mental Illness. "Mental Health Conditions." NAMI. Accessed on January 10, 2022.

Nelson, Roger (2020) "Formal Analysis September 11, 2001." The Global Consciousness Project.

Newberg, A., A. Alavi, M. Baime, M. Pourdehnad, J. Santanna, and E. d'Aquili (2001) "The Measurement of Regional Cerebral Blood Flow during the Complex Cognitive Task of Meditation: A Preliminary SPECT Study." *Psychiatry Research: Neuroimaging* 106 (2): 113–22.

Newberg, Andrew B., and Eugene G. d'Aquili (2000) "The Neuropsychology of Religious and Spiritual Experience." *Journal of Consciousness Studies* 7 (11–12): 251–66.

Newton, Michael (2010) *Destiny of Souls: New Case Studies of Life between Lives.* Woodbury, Minn.: Llewellyn Worldwide.

Northoff, G., A. Heinzel, M. De Greck, F. Bermpohl, H. Dobrowolny, and J. Panksepp (2006) "Self-Referential Processing in Our Brain: A Meta-Analysis of Imaging Studies on the Self." *Neuroimage* 31 (1): 440–57.

Öhman, Arne, Anders Flykt, and Francisco Esteves (2001) "Emotion Drives Attention: Detecting the Snake in the Grass." *Journal of Experimental Psychology: General* 130 (3): 466–78.

Open Science Collaboration (2015) "Estimating the Reproducibility of Psychological Science." *Science* 349 (6251).

Open Sciences. "The Manifesto for a Post-Materialist Science: Campaign for Open Science." Open Sciences. Accessed on April 8, 2021.

Overbye, Dennis (2021, April 7) "A Tiny Particle's Wobble Could Upend the Known Laws of Physics." *The New York Times.*

Pasricha, S., and I. Stevenson (1987) "Indian Cases of the Reincarnation Type Two Generations Apart." *Journal of the Society for Psychical Research* 54 (809): 239–246.

Persinger, Michael A. (1989) "Geophysical Variables and Behavior: LV. Predicting the Details of Visitor Experiences and the Personality of Experiments: The Temporal Lobe Factor." *Perceptual and Motor Skills* 68 (1): 55–65.

Pierre, L. S, and M. A. Persinger (2006) "Experimental Facilitation of the Sensed Presence Is Predicted by the Specific Patterns of the Applied Magnetic Fields, Not by Suggestibility: Re-Analyses of 19 Experiments." *International Journal of Neuroscience* 116 (9): 1079–96.

Pew Research Center (2009a) "Eastern, New Age Beliefs Widespread Many Americans Mix Multiple Faiths." Pew Forum.

Pew Research Center (2009b) "Religion and Science in the United States." Pew Forum.

Puthoff, Harold E., and Russell Targ (1976) "A Perceptual Channel for Information Transfer over Kilometer Distances: Historical Perspective and Recent Research." *Proceedings of the IEEE* 64 (3): 329–54.

Rabeyron, Thomas (2020) "Why Most Research Findings About Psi Are False: The Replicability Crisis, the Psi Paradox and the Myth of Sisyphus." *Frontiers in Psychology* 11 (September): 2468.

Radin, Dean (2018) *Real Magic: Ancient Wisdom, Modern Science, and a Guide to the Secret Power of the Universe*. New York: Harmony Books.

Raichle, Marcus E., Ann Mary MacLeod, Abraham Z. Snyder, William J. Powers, Debra A. Gusnard, and Gordon L. Shulman (2001) "A Default Mode of Brain Function." *Proceedings of the National Academy of Sciences of the United States of America* 98 (2): 676–82.

Raichle, M. E., and A. Z. Snyder (2007) "A Default Mode of Brain Function: A Brief History of an Evolving Idea." *Neuroimage* 37 (4): 1083–90.

Ramster, P. (1994) "Past Lives and Hypnosis." *Australian Journal of Clinical Hypnotherapy and Hypnosis* 15 (2): 67–91.

Renes, R. A., N. E. M. van Haren, H. Aarts, and M. Vink (2015) "An Exploratory fMRI Study into Inferences of Self-Agency." *Social Cognitive and Affective Neuroscience* 10 (5): 708–12.

Riba, Jordi, Peter Anderer, Francesc Jané, Bernd Saletu, and Manel J. Barbanoj (2004) "Effects of the South American Psychoactive Beverage Ayahuasca on Regional Brain Electrical Activity in Humans: A Functional Neuroimaging Study Using Low-Resolution Electromagnetic Tomography." *Neuropsychobiology* 50 (1): 89–101.

Riba, Jordi, Peter Anderer, Adelaida Morte, Gloria Urbano, Francesc Jané, Bernd Saletu, and Manel J. Barbanoj (2002) "Topographic Pharmaco-EEG Mapping of the Effects of the South American Psychoactive Beverage Ayahuasca in Healthy Volunteers." *British Journal of Clinical Pharmacology* 53 (6): 613–28.

Riccio, Matthew, Shana Cole, and Emily Balcetis (2013) "Seeing the Expected, the Desired, and the Feared: Influences on Perceptual Interpretation and Directed Attention." *Social and Personality Psychology Compass* 7 (6): 401–14.

Richard, F. D., Charles F. Bond, and Juli J. Stokes-Zoota (2003) "One Hundred Years of Social Psychology Quantitatively Described." *Review of General Psychology* 7 (4): 331–63.

Ritz, T. (2011) "Quantum Effects in Biology: Bird Navigation." *Procedia Chemistry* 1: 262–75.

Ritz, T., R. Wiltschko, P. J. Hore, C. T. Rodgers, K. Stapput, P. Thalau, C. R. Timmell, and W. Wiltschko (2009) "Magnetic Compass of Birds Is Based on a Molecule with Optimal Directional Sensitivity." *Biophysical Journal* 96 (8): 3451–57.

Rodriguez, Eugenio, Nathalie George, Jean Philippe Lachaux, Jacques Martinerie, Bernard Renault, and Francisco J. Varela (1999) "Perception's Shadow: Long-Distance Synchronization of Human Brain Activity." *Nature* 397 (6718): 430–33.

Roe, C. A, C. Sonnex, and E. C. Roxburgh (2015) "Two Meta-Analyses of Noncontact Healing Studies." *Explore* 11 (1): 11–23.

Rosenbaum, Ruth (2011) "Exploring the Other Dark Continent: Parallels between Psi Phenomena and the Psychotherapeutic Process." *Psychoanalytic Review* 98 (1): 57–90.

Rosentiel, Tom (2009) "Public Praises Science; Scientists Fault Public, Media." Pew Research.

Rouder, Jeffrey N., Richard D. Morey, and Jordan M. Province (2013) "A Bayes Factor Meta-Analysis of Recent Extrasensory Perception Experiments: Comment on Storm, Tressoldi, and Di Risio (2010)." *Psychological Bulletin* 139 (1): 241–247.

Rovelli, Carlo (1996) "Relational Quantum Mechanics." *International Journal of Theoretical Physics* 35 (8): 1637–78.

Sarraf, Matthew, Michael A. Woodley of Menie, and Patrizio Tressoldi (2020) "Anomalous Information Reception by Mediums: A Meta-Analysis of the Scientific Evidence." *Explore* 17 September-October (5): 396–402.

Satchidananda, Swami (1984) *The Yoga Sutras of Patanjali: Translation and Commentary by Sri Swami Satchidananda*. Buckingham, Va.: Integral Yoga Publications.

Schaffer, Jonathan (2009) "Spacetime the One Substance." *Philosophical Studies* 145 (1): 131–48.

Schmidt, Stefan (2015) "Experimental Research on Distant Intention Phenomena." *Parapsychology: A Handbook for the 21st Century.* Edited by Etzel Cardeña, John Palmer, and David Marcusson-Clavertz. Jefferson, N.C.: McFarland & Company, Inc.: 244–57.

Scholz, Jonathan, Christina Triantafyllou, Susan Whitfield-Gabrieli, Emery N. Brown, and Rebecca Saxe (2009) "Distinct Regions of Right Temporo-Parietal Junction Are Selective for Theory of Mind and Exogenous Attention." *PLOS One* 4 (3): e4869.

Schrödinger, Erwin (1935) "Discussion of Probability Relations Between Separated Systems," *Mathematical Proceedings of the Cambridge Philosophical Society* (31): 555–563.

Schultes, Richard Evans, and Albert Hofmann (1979) *Plants of the Gods: Origins of Hallucinogenic Use.* London: Hutchinson.

Schultes, Richard Evans, and Albert Hofmann (1992) *Plants of the Gods: Their Sacred, Healing, and Hallucinogenic Powers.* Rochester, Vt.: Healing Arts Press.

Schwarz, Katharina A., Roland Pfister, and Christian Büchel (2016) "Rethinking Explicit Expectations: Connecting Placebos, Social Cognition, and Contextual Perception." *Trends in Cognitive Sciences* 20 (6): 469-480.

Schwarz, Katharina A., Matthias J. Wieser, Antje B. M. Gerdes, Andreas Mühlberger, and Paul Pauli (2013) "Why Are You Looking like That? How the Context Influences Evaluation and Processing of Human Faces." *Social Cognitive and Affective Neuroscience* 8 (4): 438–45.

Shani, Itay (2015) "Cosmopsychism: A Holistic Approach to the Metaphysics of Experience." *Philosophical Papers* 44 (3): 389–437.

Shani, Itay, and Joachim Keppler (2018) "Beyond Combination: How Cosmic Consciousness Grounds Ordinary Experience." *Journal of the American Philosophical Association* 4 (3): 390–410.

Simons, Daniel J., and Christopher F. Chabris (1999) "Gorillas in Our Midst: Sustained Inattentional Blindness for Dynamic Events." *Perception* 28 (9): 1059–74.

Sinclair, Upton (1930) *Mental Radio.* Charlottesville, Va.: Hampton Roads Publishing Company.

Singer, Wolf, Thomas Metzinger, Johannes Gutenberg, and Jennifer M. Windt (2014) "The Ongoing Search for the Neuronal Correlate of Consciousness." Open MIND.

Smolin, Lee (1999) *The Life of the Cosmos.* Oxford: Oxford University Press.

Solov'Yov, Ilia A., Henrik Mouritsen, and Klaus Schulten (2010) "Acuity of a Cryptochrome and Vision-Based Magnetoreception System in Birds." *Biophysical journal* 99 (1): 40-49.

Steele, Claude M., and Joshua Aronson (1995) "Stereotype Threat and the Intellectual Test Performance of African Americans." *Journal of Personality and Social Psychology* 69 (5): 797–811.

Stevens, Jay (1987) *Storming Heaven: LSD and the American Dream*. New York: Grove Press.

Stevenson, Ian (1977) "The Explanatory Value of the Idea of Reincarnation." *The Journal of Nervous and Mental Disease* 164 (5): 305–26.

Stilwell, Blake (2018, April 2) "The US Military Once Successfully Used a Psychic to Locate a Lost Plane." We Are the Mighty.

Stolaroff, Myron. J. (2004) *The Secret Chief Revealed: Conversations with a Pioneer of the Underground Psychedelic Therapy Movement*. San Jose, Calif: Multidisciplinary Association for Psychedelic Studies.

Storm, Lance, and Suitbert Ertel (2001) "Does Psi Exist? Comments on Milton and Wiseman's (1999) Meta-Analysis of Ganzfield Research." *Psychological Bulletin* 127 (3): 424–33.

Storm, L., P. E. Tressoldi, and L. Di Risio (2012) "A Meta-Analysis of ESP Studies, 1987–2010: Assessing the Success of the Forced-Choice Design in Parapsychology." *Journal of Parapsychology* 76: 243–73.

Storm, Lance, Patrizio E. Tressoldi, and Lorenzo Di Risio (2010) "A Meta-Analysis With Nothing to Hide: Reply to Hyman (2010) On the Words Used to Describe Evidence for Psi." *Psychological Bulletin* 136: 491–94.

Svoboda, E., M. C. McKinnon, and B. Levine (2006) "The Functional Neuroanatomy of Autobiographical Memory: A Meta-Analysis." *Neuropsychologia* 44 (12): 2189–2208.

Tagliazucchi, Enzo, Robin Carhart-Harris, Robert Leech, David Nutt, and Dante R. Chialvo (2014) "Enhanced Repertoire of Brain Dynamical States during the Psychedelic Experience." *Human Brain Mapping* 35 (11): 5442–56.

Tagliazucchi, Enzo, Leor Roseman, Mendel Kaelen, Csaba Orban, Suresh D. Muthukumaraswamy, Kevin Murphy, Helmut Laufs, et al. (2016) "Increased Global Functional Connectivity Correlates with LSD-Induced Ego Dissolution." *Current Biology* 26 (8): 1043–50.

Tarazi, L. (1990) "An Unusual Case of Hypnotic Regression with Some Unexplained Contents." *Journal of the American Society for Psychical Research* 84 (4): 309–44.

Targ, Russell (2012) *The Reality of ESP: A Physicist's Proof of Psychic Abilities.* Wheaton, Ill: Theosophical Publishing House.

Targ, Russell (2019) "What Do We Know about Psi? The First Decade of Remote-Viewing Research and Operations at Stanford Research Institute." *Journal of Scientific Exploration* 33 (4): 569–92.

Targ, Russell, and Harold Puthoff (1974) "Information Transmission under Conditions of Sensory Shielding." *Nature* 251 (5476): 602–7.

Tarnas, Richard (2006) *Cosmos and Psyche: Intimations of a New World View.* New York: Penguin Books.

Thompson, C. (1982) "Anwesenheit: Psychopathology and Clinical Associations." *The British Journal of Psychiatry* 141 (6): 628–30.

Thurman, Michael (2016) "The Lunar Phases: Archetypes of the Soul." Mountain Astrologer.

Tracey, Irene (2010) "Getting the Pain You Expect: Mechanisms of Placebo, Nocebo and Reappraisal Effects in Humans." *Nature Medicine* 16 (11): 1277–83.

Tressoldi, Patrizio E. (2011) "Extraordinary Claims Require Extraordinary Evidence: The Case of Non-Local Perception, a Classical and Bayesian Review of Evidences." *Frontiers in Psychology* 2 (June): 117.

Tucker, Jim B. (2000) "A Scale to Measure the Strength of Children's Claims of Previous Lives: Methodology and Initial Findings." *Journal of Scientific Exploration* 14 (4): 571–81.

Turin, Luca (1996) "A Spectroscopic Mechanism for Primary Olfactory Reception." *Chemical Senses* 21 (6): 773–91.

Urgesi, Cosimo, Salvatore M. Aglioti, Miran Skrap, and Franco Fabbro (2010) "The Spiritual Brain: Selective Cortical Lesions Modulate Human Self-Transcendence." *Neuron* 65 (3).

Utts, Jessica (1996) "An Assessment of the Evidence for Psychic Functioning." *Journal of Scientific Exploration* 10 (1): 3–30.

Van Veluw, Susanne J., and Steven A. Chance (2014) "Differentiating between Self and Others: An ALE Meta-Analysis of fMRI Studies of Self-Recognition and Theory of Mind." *Brain Imaging and Behavior* 8 (March) 1: 24–38.

Vogt, B. A., and S. Laureys (2005) "Posterior Cingulate, Precuneal and Retrosplenial Cortices: Cytology and Components of the Neural Network Correlates of Consciousness." *Progress in Brain Research* (150): 205–17.

Vollenweider, Franz X., and Mark A. Geyer (2001) "A Systems Model of Altered

Consciousness: Integrating Natural and Drug-Induced Psychoses." *Brain Research Bulletin* 56 (November) 5: 495–507.

Vollenweider, F. X., K. L. Leenders, C. Scharfetter, P. Maguire, O. Stadelmann, and J. Angst (1997) "Positron Emission Tomography and Fluorodeoxyglucose Studies of Metabolic Hyperfrontality and Psychopathology in the Psilocybin Model of Psychosis." *Neuropsychopharmacology* 16 (5): 357–72.

Voss, Joel L., Carol L. Baym, and Ken A. Paller (2008) "Accurate Forced-Choice Recognition without Awareness of Memory Retrieval." *Learning and Memory* 15 (6): 454–59.

Voss, Joel L., Heather D. Lucas, and Ken A. Paller (2012) "More than a Feeling: Pervasive Influences of Memory without Awareness of Retrieval." *Cognitive Neuroscience* 3 (3–4): 193–207.

Wahbeh, Helané, Dean Radin, Julia Mossbridge, Cassandra Vieten, and Arnaud Delorme (2018) "Exceptional Experiences Reported by Scientists and Engineers." *Explore* 14 (5): 329–41.

Wasson, R. Gordon, and Valentina Pavlovna Wasson (1957) *Mushrooms, Russia, and History.* 2 vols. New York: Pantheon.

Watt, Caroline, and Marleen Nagtegaal (2004) "Reporting of Blind Methods: An Interdisciplinary Survey." *Journal of the Society for Psychical Research, 68* (875)[2]: 105–14.

Webber, John (2020) *The Red Chair.* Carlsbad, Calif: Balboa Press.

Weil, Gunther M., Ralph Metzner, and Timothy Leary, eds. (1965) *The Psychedelic Reader.* New York: University Books.

Weiss, Brian L. (1988) *Many Lives, Many Masters.* New York: Fireside Books.

Weiss, Brian L. (1992) *Through Time Into Healing.* New York: Fireside Books.

Wheeler, John Archibald (1973) "From Relativity to Mutability." *The Physicist's Conception of Nature.* Dordrecht, Neth: Springer: 202–47

Williams, B. J. (2011) "Revisiting the Ganzfeld ESP Debate: A Basic Review and Assessment." *Journal of Scientific Exploration* 25 (4): 639–undefined.

Yaden, David B., and Roland R. Griffiths (2021) "The Subjective Effects of Psychedelics Are Necessary for Their Enduring Therapeutic Effects." *ACS Pharmacology and Translational Science* 4 (2), 568–72.

Zdrenka, Marco, and Marc S. Wilson (2017) "Individual Difference Correlates of Psi Performance in Forced-Choice Precognition Experiments: A Meta-Analysis (1945–2016)." *The Journal of Parapsychology* 81 (1): 9–32.

# Index

Page numbers in *italics* refer to illustrations.

of senility and lead to a false diagnosis of Alzheimer's disease. Senile dementia is attributable to end-stage syphilis, the syphilitic diathesis within homeopathy, and environmental toxicity. It may also result from the abominations of animal husbandry.[14]

Prions, or "proteinaceous infectious particles," are peculiar and unique disease-causing proteins, found by the neurologist Stanley B. Prusiner in the early 1980s; Prusiner called the protein PrP, for "prion protein." For reasons and by means as yet unknown, prions are able to invert their structure, replicate, and change their shape, converting normal protein molecules into dangerous ones. Also called spongiform encephalopathies, prion diseases are fatal: the proliferation of prions leaves gaping holes in the brain tissue of mammals. The most common form, found in sheep and goats, is called *scrapie,* a term arising from the animals' need to scrape off their wool or hair because of an intense symptomatic itch. Bovine spongiform encephalopathy, named Mad Cow disease, was identified in cows in Great Britain in 1986; the source of the disease was found to be a food supplement fed to the cows made from *ground-up carcasses of cattle and sheep,* which may have been infected with a brain-wasting disease.

When foisting a carnivorous and cannibalistic diet on vegetarian cattle our species shows disdain for the Great Circle of Life containing cattle and all other animals. Scorn of our humble position within nature's kingdom is spiritual loss of reference. My conjecture is that consuming meat from abominably treated cattle ushers us into madness: Alzheimer's disease with its characteristic loss of reference.

**shell shock.** See *post-traumatic stress disorder.*

**sinfulness as a diathesis.** Religion perceives this as madness due to having strayed from God, of having forsaken a moral obligation to offset the state of original sinfulness to which, due to Adam's eating of the apple, we are heir. The masturbation thesis of madness denotes an activity offensive to God. (See also *masturbatory madness.*)

**sociopath.** A sociopath can be defined as a psychopath with a weak rather than an absent conscience. Within the materia medica of the remedy Anacardium orientale, cruelty and struggle within the conscience— akin to a battle between one's "good" and one's "bad" angels—is described. I have speculated that the Unabomber, Theodore Kaczynski, could have been helped by this remedy.

**Stockholm syndrome.** A syndrome named after a hostage situation in Stockholm in 1973, in which four bank employees bonded with their captors, sided with them against police, and defended them later in court. Psychologists believe that this tendency to identify with someone who is actually abusive, threatening, or dangerous is a coping mechanism in a situation when the victim cannot escape. Stockholm syndrome can also be acquired in consequence of one's having experienced long-term abuse. Constitutional remedy states can reflect a mirroring of trauma's effects. In addition to predisposing us to ailments such as head pain, we find as with any acute emergency that chronic emotional states register—but also directly mirror—psychic trauma. As an example, the psyche of an individual subjected to long-standing belittlement by his parents comes to buy their argument that he is inferior, worthless, stupid, or incompetent. As in Stockholm syndrome he has adopted as his own the perspective of his oppressors. In a case such as this the constitutional remedy Thuja is often prescribed. When the mirroring involves adoption of an ideology the individual is said to be brainwashed.

**suicidal.** Though not a specific diagnosis within psychiatry, suicidal thinking is considered symptomatic of other conditions, such as depression or borderline personality. Within ancient Greek myths it was an understandable, sometimes even necessary solution to intense psychological suffering. Within the German Sturm und Drang movement of the late eighteenth century, as displayed in Goethe's *The Sorrows of Young Werther* (in this case a young man's extreme response to unrequited love), it is a beautiful release from excess of emotion not reconcilable by reason. Within a non-individualistically oriented society such as Japan's ancient samurai warrior class, it was called for on the part of an individual who may not have been personally responsible for a catastrophe but must perform ritual suicide (*seppuku*) so that harmony within the social structure could be reestablished. This brings to mind the homeopathic remedy Naja.

**sycotic diathesis.** Due to familial or inherited legacy of gonorrhea, a susceptibility to depersonalization, monomania, recklessness, guilt, and self-torment. Discussed in chapter 9. Traditional Chinese medicine utilizes a schema known as the Five Phases that superficially bears similarity to the Four Humors. Accordingly, in TCM a manic, overly sanguine individual might be diagnosed as suffering from an excess of heart yang (fire), whereas a choleric individual might be diagnosed as suffering from liver wind (wood), a phlegmatic individual could be diagnosed as spleen-qi deficient (earth), a panic-stricken individual with a kidney deficiency (water).

**syphilitic diathesis.** Due to familial or an inherited legacy of this sexually transmitted disease, a susceptibility to paranoia, addictiveness, obsessiveness, circular thinking, and tissue breakdown. Discussed in chapter 7.

**syphilitic insanity.** Paralytic dementia due to late-stage syphilis. (See also *senile dementia*.)

**Tourette's syndrome.** A disorder that can include coprolalia (involuntary, repetitive use of obscene language) and repetitive movements that can't be easily controlled, such as eye blinking, shoulder shrugging, or blurting out unusual sounds. Much more often seen among boys than girls, it is responsive to remedies such as Anacardium and Tarentula hispanica.

**tubercular diathesis.** Due to familial or an inherited legacy of tuberculosis, manifests as a susceptibility to extremes of yearning, restlessness, frenzy, and religious- and grief-inspired mania.

**warning out.** In the early nineteenth century, individuals with disabilities and others considered deviant were often "warned out," meaning, for example, informed upon when the poor-soul newcomer was unwelcome in town. A dire next step of warning out was "passing on," loading such persons onto a cart and dropping them off in the next town. American cities today regularly offer one-way bus tickets out of town to homeless persons, many of whom suffer from mental illness. In Los Angeles, buses carrying recently freed prisoners have been observed disgorging them onto Skid Row. Where shall they dwell?

**wise man.** Pertaining to the Renaissance in accordance with a theory of Michel Foucault's. According to Foucault the mad were then portrayed in art as possessing wisdom—knowledge of the limits of our world. A modern example would be the broadcaster character Howard Beale from the 1976 comedy-drama film *Network,* written by Paddy Chayefsky. Beale's denunciation of societal dehumanization was prescient but viewed as crazed by the authoritarian forces he was indicting.

------------------------

# Exemplifying Nanomedicine: The Research of Dr. Iris Bell

September 18, 2015, saw delivery of a momentous verdict.

A putative class of plaintiffs seeking $250 million in damages had sued Hylands, Inc., and the Standard Homeopathic Company for falsely and misleadingly representing the effectiveness of active ingredients in homeopathic products. Brief deliberation in federal court resulted in exoneration of the defendants, who were found not in breach of any express warranty or violation of the California Consumer Legal Remedies Act.[1]

While signaling an endorsement of homeopathic medicine, repudiation of the plaintiff's allegations also dealt a blow to the pharmaceutical industry's anti-homeopathy campaign. The jury's reckoning that homeopathic medicine rests on established science is reverberating within the health care industry.

For this we can thank Dr. Iris Bell. A former Harvard psychiatry instructor and holder of a doctorate from Stanford University in neuro- and biobehavioral sciences, Dr. Bell had consulted with Highlands, Inc., to design the company's clinical trials. Dr. Bell's testimony about state-of-the-art nanomedicine within her area of expertise, multiple chemical sensitivity and homeopathy, was the deciding factor.

Dr. Bell's supporting paper terms her concept "Adaptive Network

Nanomedicine: An Integrated Model for Homeopathic Medicine."[2] In brief, this refers to minuscule entities known as nanoparticles and nanobubbles shown to have an effect on biological cells in low doses, creating hormetic effects. *Hormesis,* a term used by toxicologists to describe an organism's adaptation to stimuli, describes a biphasic (two-phased) response to an external agent in varying dosages. In an initial phase low-dose stimulation is pleasing or beneficial. In a second phase response, increased dosage or more frequent stimulation from the same agent produces an inhibitory or toxic effect.

In parallel with my concept of radical disjunct, hormesis in simple terms means getting too much of any good thing is bad. We know that eating is necessary to health (phase one), whereas overeating (phase two) is bad. Similarly, exercise is beneficial, physical overwork is not; the mini-stabbing of acupuncture needles is medicinal, being stabbed with a knife is not. Continuous dosage invites medication overexposure. Is this surprising? The principle of hormesis says, hardly!

Poisoning, meaning exposure to a gross amount of a toxic substance, can be lethal. Regardless of its toxicology text portrayal, in the right circumstance and for a particular individual, micro-dosage exposure to the same noxious substance is nanomedicine, indicating homeopathy. It is as a prescient Zen master Unmon said: "Illness and medicine cure one another. Where does one find the self?"

Beyond the two-phase two step, hormesis figures into a familiar feedback loop that we term stress relief. Normal functioning finds homeostasis perpetually lost, regained, lost, and regained again. The toggling between pleasing and non-pleasing effects, irritation and relief, the buildup of tension and tension release is known as allostasis.

## HOMEOPATHY FACILITATES ALLOSTASIS

To date a variety of theories have been proposed to explain homeopathic remedy effects. These include

- persistent memory of unique water structures,[3]
- water-ethanol clusters and nanobubbles,[4]

- epitaxy and glass-derived silica crystals and structures,[5]
- electromagnetic activities (Dr. Bell),[6]
- biological signaling (Dr. Bell),[7] and
- quantum macro entanglement.[8]

Dr. Bell's nanoparticle–cross adaptation–sensitization model incorporates and builds upon conceptual points and empirical findings from this prior body of work. In keeping with common homeopathic practice, Dr. Bell's hormetic effects reflect intermittent, low-dosage prescribing, the effect of which is stage-by-stage nanoparticle processing within the biological system culminating in a global summary response. Her concept of nanoparticle–cross adaptation–sensitization is charted below:

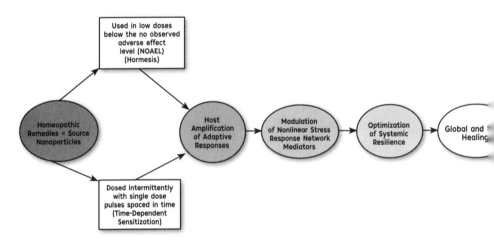

**Nanoparticle–cross adaptation–sensitization**
Based on Bell and Koithan, "A Model for Homeopathic Remedy Effects," figure 1

## THE NONLINEAR ALLOSTATIC STRESS RESPONSE NETWORK (NASRN)

What we think of as the mind actually involves the whole body. A question for the ages opposes reductionism to vitalism: Is the mind reducible to the physiological activity in the brain, or is the mind vital, a separate and independent entity? Put another way, if we liken the brain to a soup cooking in the kitchen, does the soup cook itself?

Homeopaths maintain that the soup does not cook itself. A separate and independent entity underlying consciousness, known as the vital force, is the chef. We can think of the vital force as a subconscious imbued with physiological awareness, function, and the wherewithal to respond to stress.

From this standpoint reductionist biological models, though wonderfully descriptive, are not really explanatory. The model at hand presenting the players in drama of stress is a bridge between the realms of vitalism and reductionism.

In response to stress, two-way communication between the brain and the cardiovascular, immune, and other systems via neural and endocrine mechanisms occurs that either promotes or reflects the movement of consciousness. These interactions express our individualized stress and our individual susceptibility to disease. Stressful events need not be overly dramatic. They can involve events of normal daily life that impact physiological activities such as sleep, metabolism, and anything leading to a stressed-out feeling.

The incremental toll this takes on the body, called "allostatic load," reflects not only the effect of life events but also of epigenetic pressures due to lifestyle: ingrained patterns relating to diet, exercise, and substance abuse, for example. Hormones afford the body short-term protection and promote more established adaptation (learning), but in the long run allostatic load causes changes in the body that can lead to disease. It is in the brain that levels of stress are ascertained, allostasis regulated, and allostatic load assessed. This occurs in regions such as the hippocampus, amygdala, and prefrontal cortex, all of which respond to acute and chronic stress by undergoing structural remodeling, which alters behavioral and physiological responses. The network of their interaction can be modeled as in the following diagram (see page 214).

Elemental stressors and nanoparticle ameliorators to the NASRN do not act upon a blank slate. Within biological systems the preexisting terrain of individuated, cognitive, and emotional tendencies is an animating force, what in ordinary terms we know of as consciousness.[9]

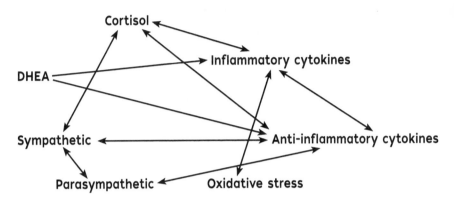

**Stress Adaptive Network**
Based on Bell and Koithan, "A Model for Homeopathic
Remedy Effects," figure 2

## ACTORS IN THE PHYSIOLOGICAL
## DRAMA OF STRESS

*The following discussion draws extensively on Zhang and An's article "Cytokines, Inflammation and Pain."*

The amygdala coordinates behavioral, autonomic, and endocrine responses suffused with emotional content. The hippocampus helps control corticosteroid production but while doing so actively encodes and retrieves memories. The orbital frontal cortex, critical to judgment, insight, motivation, and mood, engineers depression when functioning abnormally. Following are some physiological components of this terrain.

- *Parasympathetic autonomic nervous system.* The parasympathetic nervous system (PNS) and sympathetic nervous system (SNS) are both part of the autonomic nervous system responsible for the body's involuntary functions. Located between the spinal cord and the medulla, the PNS predominates in the body's "rest and digest" and "feed and breed" responses. It regulates the heart rate, respiration, pupillary response, and more. The SNS activates a "fight or flight" response to a perceived threat. The PNS restores the body to a state of calm.

- *Inflammatory cytokines.* "Inflammatory responses in the peripheral and central nervous systems play key roles in the development and persistence of many pathological pain states. Certain inflammatory cytokines in the spinal cord, dorsal root ganglion (DRG) of a spinal nerve, and injured nerve or skin are known to be associated with pain behaviors and with the generation of abnormal spontaneous activity from injured nerve fibers or compressed/inflamed DRG neurons."[10]

- *"Cytokines* are small, secreted proteins released by cells that have a specific effect on the interactions and communications between cells. Cytokine is a general name; other names include lymphokine (cytokines made by lymphocytes), monokine (cytokines made by monocytes), chemokine (cytokines with chemotactic activities), and interleukin (cytokines made by one leukocyte and acting on other leukocytes). Cytokines may act on the cells that secrete them (autocrine action), on nearby cells (paracrine action), or in some instances on distant cells (endocrine action)."[11]

- *"Anti-inflammatory cytokines* are a series of immunoregulatory molecules that control the pro-inflammatory cytokine response. Cytokines act in concert with specific cytokine inhibitors and soluble cytokine receptors to regulate the human immune response. Their physiologic role in inflammation and pathologic role in systemic inflammatory states are increasingly recognized."[12]

- *DHEA.* An important precursor hormone, dehydroepiandrosterone is the highest circulating steroid present in the human body. It has scant biological effect on its own but is powerful when converted into hormones such as testosterone and estradiol. DHEA is produced from cholesterol by the outer layer of the adrenal glands and in small amounts by the ovary and testes. An important source of estrogen for women, DHEA production gradually increases from age ten, peaks during the twenties, and decreases with aging.[13]

- *Cortisol.* A steroid hormone, one of the glucocorticoids, cortisol is made in the cortex of the adrenal glands and then released into the blood, which transports it throughout the body. Almost every cell contains receptors for cortisol, so cortisol can have numerous actions depending on the type of cell receiving it. These effects include regulating blood sugar level, anti-inflammatory activity, memory sustaining or conversely loss of recall, controlling salt and water balance, regulating blood pressure, and is a factor in development of a fetus.

- *Oxidative stress.* The phenomenon of stress results from the imbalance of "production and accumulation of oxygen reactive species (ROS) in cells and tissues and the ability of a biological system to detoxify these reactive products." As ROS plays various cell-signaling roles and are normally by-products of oxygen metabolism, they are subject to environmental stressors (that is, UV, ionizing radiations, pollutants, and heavy metals) and xenobiotics (antiblastic drugs). When such stressors contribute to the increased ROS production, the resulting imbalance leads to cell and tissue damage that we term oxidative stress.[14]

Were the outputs of these functions quantifiable, schematic depiction of an individual's characteristic stresses and tensions would emerge. If the outputs could be depicted dynamically, an animation of the vital force in a state of health or reflective of illness susceptibility could result.

## REGULATING THE BIOLOGICAL SYSTEM

Dr. Bell's model explains pathogenesis: Accumulating stress overwhelms a biological system's capacity to adapt. Dysregulation results.

The detoxifying experience that is acute illness requires allostasis to intensify. Fever and inflammation arise and culminate before homeostasis is restored. Whereas an acute crisis eventuates in robust homeostasis, chronic illness exhibits compromised homeostasis. As symptoms are permitted to linger, mental, emotional, and physical polarities arise; and susceptibility to illness proliferates.

Chronic illness involves diminishment of hormesis and compromised capacity to adapt. In place of battling for homeostasis, a dysregulated system appeases the toxins and stressors it confronts. Defeatist terms are agreed to as the biological system grants resident status to the dysregulated state's worst features.

According to Dr. Bell and Mary Koithan, the problem is surmountable. "Targeted, timed disruption of the dysfunctional dynamics of disease affords the system an opportunity to recover normal regulatory relationships and interactions across the biological network."[15] What Bell and Koithan are describing is a method that exemplifies nanomedicine—namely, homeopathy.

# APPENDIX 3

---

# Samuel Hahnemann's Mental Health Aphorisms

Samuel Hahnemann went to great lengths to deny mental ailments their own diagnostic category. This is not to say he took the problem lightly. Quite the contrary. His position, as stated in aphorism 216, was that such disorders "can only be detected by the observation of a physician gifted with perseverance and penetration." Moreover, the language he used when referring to mental unbalance was, as in the following examples, unstintingly vivid: "derangement of the mind and disposition" (aphorism 215); "a real moral or mental malady" (aphorism 224); "furious mania . . . doleful, querulous lamentation . . . senseless chattering . . . disgusting and abominable conduct" (aphorism 224).[1]

So that his ideas could be expressed logically and succinctly, Samuel Hahnemann wrote his renowned work, the *Organon of the Healing Art* (earlier titled *The Organon of the Rational Healing Science*), in aphoristic style (paragraphs with numbering). The book went through six editions in all, with five editions published during Hahnemann's lifetime. The sixth edition was completed in 1842, but as he passed away before it could be published, it was not printed until 1921, when Dr. William Boericke, known today as the compiler and editor of the *Pocket Manual of Homeopathic Materia Medica,* brought it to light. As the prose can be dense, I have ventured to summarize the key ideas.

## ORGANON APHORISM §210

*Of psoric origin are almost all those diseases that I have above termed one-sided, which appear to be more difficult to cure in consequence of this one-sidedness, all their other morbid symptoms disappearing, as it were, before the single, great, prominent symptom. Of this character are what are termed "mental diseases." They do not, however, constitute a class of disease sharply separated from all others, since in all other so-called corporeal diseases the condition of the disposition and mind is* always *altered; and in all cases of disease we are called on to cure the state of the patient's disposition is to be particularly noted, along with the totality of the symptoms, if we would trace an accurate picture of the disease, in order to be able therefrom to treat it homeopathically with success.*

### Commentary

*Psoric* refers to what Hahnemann considered a miasm (residual effects of disease in an individual's lineage), in this case a primordial miasm preceding all other miasms, *psora*. Designated the "itch," it has been proposed that psora relates to epigenetically established candida. In practice suppression of the primordial itch reveals an existential issue related to poor adjustment to happenstance, a mild version of which is normal. Aligning himself with allopathic medical colleagues, Talcott invariably eschewed use of the psoric term, preferring the more recognizable *diathesis* whenever referring to miasma.

By *one-sided* Hahnemann is saying that the preponderance of mental symptoms in relation to physical symptoms make mental conditions hard to cure, though at the same time, mental conditions do not constitute a separate domain of illness since, as with all patients, the totality of symptoms determines the treatment and remedy choice.

## ORGANON APHORISM §211

*This holds good to such an extent, that the state of the disposition of the patient often chiefly determines the selection of the homeopathic remedy, as being a decidedly characteristic symptom which can least of all remain concealed from the accurately observing physician.*

### Commentary

Hahnemann is urging the physician to attend to something obvious, the strangest, least common mental or emotional feature the patient displays. This characteristic symptom provides a key clue for remedy selection.

## ORGANON APHORISM §212

*The Creator of therapeutic agents has also had particular regard to this main feature of all diseases, the altered state of the disposition and mind, for there is no powerful medicinal substance in the world which does not very notably alter the state of the disposition and mind in the healthy individual who tests it, and every medicine does so in a different manner.*

### Commentary

Hahnemann is paralleling the uniqueness of the unlimited forms mental dispositions can take with the variety of ways medicinals can alter mental disposition.

## ORGANON APHORISM §213

*We shall, therefore, never be able to cure conformably to nature—that is to say, homeopathically—if we do not, in every case of disease, even in such as are acute, observe, along with the other symptoms, those relating to the changes in the state of the mind and disposition; and if we do not select, for the patient's relief, from among the medicines a disease-force, which in addition to the similarity of its other symptoms to those of the disease, is also capable of producing a similar state of the disposition and mind.*

### Commentary

Whether a condition be acute or chronic, it cannot be cured other than by recourse to the Law of Similars.

## ORGANON APHORISM §214

*The instructions I have to give relative to the cure of mental diseases may be confined to a very few remarks, as they are to be cured in the same way as all other diseases, namely, by a remedy which shows, by the symptoms it causes in the body and mind of a healthy individual, a power of producing a morbid state as similar as possible to the case of disease before us, and in no other way can they be cured.*

### *Commentary*
Mental conditions are cured just as any other conditions are cured, according to how the remedy is researched homeopathically via provings (see appendix 1) in healthy people.

## ORGANON APHORISM §215

*Almost all the so-called mental and emotional diseases are nothing more than corporeal diseases in which the symptom of derangement of the mind and disposition peculiar to each of them is increased, whilst the corporeal symptoms decline (more or less rapidly), till it at length attains the most striking one-sidedness, almost as though it were a local disease in the invisible subtle organ of the mind or disposition.*

### *Commentary*
In a worsening mental/emotional state the physical symptoms can be seen to decline proportionately, but this is not good as the case's one-sidedness makes it more difficult to cure. Though not a physical entity it is as though the mind is an organ, albeit an invisible, subtle one.

## ORGANON APHORISM §216

*The cases are not rare in which a so-called corporeal disease that threatens to be fatal—a suppuration of the lungs, or the deterioration of some other important viscus, or some other disease of acute character, e.g., in childbed, etc.—becomes transformed into insanity, into a kind of melancholia or into mania by a rapid increase of the psychical symptoms that were previously present, whereupon the corporeal symptoms lose all their danger; these latter improve almost to perfect health, or rather they decrease to such a degree that their obscured presence can only be detected by the observation of a physician gifted with perseverance and penetration. In this manner they become transformed into a one-sided and, as if it were, a local disease, in which the symptom of the mental disturbance, which was at first but slight, increases so as to be the chief symptom, and in a great measure occupies the place of the other (corporeal) symptoms, whose intensity it subdues in a palliative manner, so that, in short, the affections of the grosser corporeal organs become, as it were, transferred and conducted to the almost spiritual mental and emotional organs, which the anatomist has never yet and never will reach with his scalpel.*

## Commentary

This is an elaboration on aphorism 215. Examples are provided where the physical presentation improves as the mind deteriorates. The skill of an experienced physician is needed so that the source of the mental deterioration within physiological pathology may be located. Even so, the problem at this level is impervious to cure by surgical means.

## ORGANON APHORISM §221

*If, however, insanity or mania (caused by fright, vexation, the abuse of spirituous liquors, etc.) have suddenly broken out as an acute disease in the patient's ordinary calm state, although it almost always arises from internal psora, like a flame bursting forth from it, yet when it occurs in this acute manner it should not be immediately treated with antipsorics, but in the first place with remedies indicated for it out of the other class of proved medicaments (e.g., Aconite, Belladonna, Stramonium, Hyoscyamus, Mercury, etc.) in highly potentized, minute, homeopathic doses, in order to subdue it so far that the psora shall for the time revert to its former latent state, wherein the patient appears as if quite well.*

## Commentary

If the breakout of madness is due to recent causes it should be treated as an acute condition. Rather than deal with an underlying existential (psoric) issue, use familiar remedies to return the patient to his baseline state. This is a principle adhered to in sane asylums.

## ORGANON APHORISM §224

*If the mental disease be not quite developed, and if it be still somewhat doubtful whether it really arose from a corporeal affection, or did not rather result from faults of education, bad practices, corrupt morals, neglect of the mind, superstition, or ignorance; the mode of deciding this point will be, that if it proceed from one or other of the latter causes it will diminish and be improved by sensible friendly exhortations, consolatory arguments, serious representations, and sensible advice; whereas a real moral or mental malady, depending on bodily disease, would be speedily aggravated by such a course, the melancholic would become still more dejected, querulous, inconsolable, and reserved, the spiteful maniac would thereby become still more exasperated, and the chattering fool would become manifestly more foolish.*

## Commentary

The more serious forms of madness are rooted in physiology, but that is not easy to discern. Morality or lifestyle-augmenting therapies will help the non-physiologically based cases. But they will worsen cases that are physiologically rooted (and which call for accurate homeopathy).

## ORGANON APHORISM §228

*In mental and emotional diseases resulting from corporeal maladies, which can only be cured by homeopathic antipsoric medicine conjoined with carefully regulated mode of life, an appropriate psychical behavior toward the patient on the part of those about him and of the physician must be scrupulously observed, by way of an auxiliary mental regimen. To furious mania we must oppose calm intrepidity and cool, firm resolution; to doleful, querulous lamentation, a mute display of commiseration in looks and gestures; to senseless chattering, a silence not wholly inattentive; to disgusting and abominable conduct and to conversation of a similar character, total inattention. We must merely endeavor to prevent the destruction and injury of surrounding objects, without reproaching the patient for his acts, and everything must be arranged in such a way that the necessity for any corporeal punishments and tortures whatever may be avoided. This is so much the more easily effected because in the administration of the medicine—the only circumstance in which the employment of coercion could be justified—in the homeopathic system the small doses of the appropriate medicine never offend the taste, and may consequently be given to the patient without his knowledge in his drink, so that all compulsion is unnecessary.*

### Commentary

Hahnemann is describing an ideal and compassionate manner in which the mentally ill should be approached. He says that the only time coercion is justified involves the necessary administration of a homeopathic medicine that in any case is minuscule and neither bad tasting nor detectable. How this works out in actual practice is best described in Clara Barrus's text, *Nursing the Insane*.

# ORGANON APHORISM §229

*On the other hand, contradiction, eager explanations, rude corrections, and invectives, as also weak, timorous yielding are quite out of place with such patients; they are equally pernicious modes of treating mental and emotional maladies. But such patients are most of all exasperated and their complaint aggravated by contumely, fraud, and deceptions that they can detect. The physician and keeper must always pretend to believe them to be possessed of reason.*

*All kinds of external disturbing influences on their senses and disposition should be if possible removed; there are no amusements for their clouded spirit, no salutary distractions, no means of instruction, no soothing effects from conversation, books, or other things for the soul that pines or frets in the chains of the diseased body, no invigoration for it but the cure; it is only when the bodily health is changed for the better that tranquility and comfort again beam upon their mind.*

## Commentary

Hahnemann is advising caregivers to invest themselves in a belief that the patient possesses the capacity to recover reason. This means acting as if they believe and take seriously whatever the patient says. As the patient is far more likely to improve in an atmosphere of tranquillity, he also insists on the removal of distractive amusements.

---------------------------

# Middletown State Homeopathic Hospital Treatments and Case Studies

As conditions meriting special attention, Talcott's *Mental Diseases and Their Modern Treatment* targets melancholia, mania, dementia, and paresis. The materia medica of remedies he provides at the end of the book reflect these areas of interest. To encounter the medicines' application in actual cases treated at the Middletown Hospital we have recourse to the *Twenty-Fourth Annual Report of the Middletown State Homeopathic Hospital*. In the second part of this chapter, "A Sampling of Case Records," I provide these cases verbatim in the order they are given in the 1895 report.

## MEDICAL TREATMENTS

The following excerpts are from Talcott's *Mental Diseases and Their Modern Treatment*.

### *Melancholia*

*Let us now turn our attention to a few remedies for melancholia. It has long been supposed that Aurum metallicum was a princely remedy for suicidal melancholia. Our experience has not sustained this theory. Aurum has often been prescribed in apparently indicated cases, but usually without good effects. We have a remedy in the Materia Medica which has worked very satisfactorily in cases of restless, resistive, agitated and suicidal melancholia, and that remedy is Arsenicum.*

*The patients that Arsenicum has relieved have been those whose physical condition would naturally suggest the administration of that drug. These patients have been much emaciated, and have had wretched appetites. They present a dry, red, tremulous tongue; they exhibit a shriveled skin, and a haggard and anxious countenance. They look as if they had suffered the tortures of the damned, and that the fiends of hell were still getting in their fine work. The Arsenicum case is very thirsty, but is easily satisfied with a small quantity. The Arsenicum patient is not only inclined to wear himself out by constant exercise, but he is likewise inclined to kill himself, or, failing in that, he is apt to mutilate the body by chewing the fingers, by pulling out the eyelids, by scratching holes in the face and scalp, and by torturing the flesh generally.*

*For acute melancholia, where the victim is prostrated by shock, where the grief is intensely profound, where the power of weeping, and thus securing relief, has been abolished, there we find Ignatia amara the relieving remedy. Probably no drug has produced more comforting results in the realms of sorrow and of loss than the St. Ignatius bean. The Ignatia patient wants to be left alone, and is yet sensitive about what she conceives to be the neglect of her friends. For brooding sorrow, following hard luck or bad news, give Ignatia. For the overmastering effects of good news, which impel some women into the hysteric state, give Coffea. While the Ignatia patient generally broods, she sometimes becomes hysterical, and indulges in temporary fits of laughter.*

*The Natrum muriaticum patients, instead of brooding over their troubles or crying inwardly (Ignatia), bubble and shed tears copiously like the old prince and king over their alleged dead brother, as described in* Huckleberry Finn. *The more you attempt to quiet them, the more effusively they weep. If contradicted, they become ill-humored and easily provoked, like Chamomilla and Bryonia. Natrum muriaticum patients are generally thin and anemic, and have a prematurely old age appearance. This remedy is often indicated in cases of melancholia following intermittent fever, and when the patients have periodic attacks of violent weeping.*

*Among the crybaby remedies we have Pulsatilla, Nux moschata, and Cactus. The Pulsatilla patient weeps easily, but smiles through her tears and is very changeable. The mental state of Pulsatilla is like the weather in April—now you see the brilliant radiance of the summer's sun as it glints down from cerulean-hued heavens; and again, you see gray skies, or feel the trickling tears of the clouds.*

*The Cactus patient is sad and hypochondriacal; not inclined to speak; weeps quietly but steadily. And for accompanying symptoms there are marked palpitations of the heart, with heavy pressure in the head as if a weight lay on the vertex, and pulsations in the top of the head.*

*Nux moschata is a remedy for a melancholy person with hysterical tendencies. The mood is changeable; one moment the patient laughs, and the next cries. Mental activity under Nux moschata is greatly depressed. The ideas are confused, more so than in Pulsatilla, and there is an inability to continue a train of thought for any length of time. There is loss of memory, and a stupid condition like Anacardium, Opium, and Phosphoric acid. In speaking or writing, Nux moschata patients are given to dreamy incoherence of expression.*

*Digitalis is a remedy that is useful in melancholia with stupor, or in any depressed state when the pulse is slow, and the general circulation throughout the system very stagnant, and when the eyes seem to be brimming with tears.*

*Gelsemium is called for in melancholia when there is much fever, a general dullness of the mental faculties, and a desire to lie in bed and be let alone.*

*Opium is sometimes used in chronic melancholia when there is vivid imagination, and when the patients are easily frightened; or when there are marked stupidity and hopelessness, with contraction of the pupils.*

*Veratrum album is called for in melancholia when physical prostration and mental hopelessness follow an outbreak of maniacal excitement.*

*Actea racemosa, Lilium tigrinum, and Sepia are important remedies in the treatment of melancholic women who are suffering with ovarian or uterine troubles. The mental depression in such cases seems to arise from an abnormal condition of the generative organs. Both Lilium and Sepia are full of apprehensions, and manifest much anxiety for their welfare. In the Sepia case, however, there is likely to be found some serious change in the* uterine organs, while the Lilium case presents either functional disturbance, or comparatively superficial organic lesion. Lilium is more applicable to acute cases of melancholia when the uterus or ovaries are involved in moderate inflammation, and when the patient apprehends the presence of a fatal disease which does not exist.

The Lilium case quite speedily recovers, much to her own surprise, as well as that of her friends. The Sepia patient is despairing, somewhat suicidal, and averse to work or exercise. This remedy is called for most frequently in cases of long-continued uterine disorder and consequent mental depression.

Actea racemosa acts in a more general and less specific manner than either Lilium or Sepia. The entire nervous system is affected by the use of Actea, and the condition produced is that of a depressing irritant. The female sexual organs are profoundly impressed by this drug. The menses become erratic and delayed. At the same time the patient feels as if her mind were wrapped in a deep black cloud. She also feels as if she were going crazy, and as if death were impending. Intense mental depression, with spasmodic seizures during menstruation, headache in the back of the head, extending over the neck, with rheumatic pains in the muscles of the neck and back, are some of the indications for Actea in melancholia.

## Mania

We will now consider a few remedies which have been used successfully for the cure of mania; and, first of all, we will present that medical "Old Guard" composed of the "Big Four" therapeutic veterans—namely, Belladonna, Hyoscyamus, Stramonium, and Veratrum album.

No remedy in the Materia Medica possesses a wider range of action, or a greater power for relieving distressing symptoms in the brain than Belladonna. Its symptoms are clear and well defined. Its action is sharp, vigorous, and profound. It is a powerful supplementary ally of Aconite in clearing away the last vestige of cerebral congestion; and beyond this it subdues effectively the subtle processes of inflammation. Its symptoms are familiar to every student of Materia Medica, but it may be well to state, just here, that in a case of insanity where Belladonna is indicated you will find a hot, flushed face (the face is bright red throughout), dilated pupils, throbbing arteries, a fixed and savage look, with now and then sudden spasmodic ebullitions of rage and fury.

*The Belladonna patient tosses in vague uncertain restlessness. He attempts to bite, strike, tear clothes, strip off clothing, and make outrageous exhibitions of the person, not on account of lecherousness like Cantharis, but because of a disposition to destroy everything that is reachable or tearable. The Belladonna patients are exceedingly fickle, and constantly changing in their mental states. They change suddenly from one mood to another, sing, and laugh for a short time. But all their moods end in a cyclonic outburst of violence and intolerable rage. Belladonna produces these conditions and symptoms when taken in material doses, and it has relieved, and probably cured, many a case of insanity.*

*There are two rather opposite conditions existing under the influence of Belladonna. In overpowering doses the Belladonna patient, after the first period of excitement, becomes dull and heavy, with stertorous breathing, and dark-red besotted countenance, somewhat similar to that of Gelsemium.*

*On the other hand, we find other Belladonna cases exceedingly excitable and nervous, and inclined to move all the time. These are the extreme effects of Belladonna, either a stupid, apoplectic condition on the one hand, and on the other the light, loquacious, active, excited, and restless state of mind. The excitable patient will become quiet under small doses of Belladonna—that is, from the third to the thirtieth potencies, while the stupid patient seems to require a large dose—that is, the first centesimal, or even the first decimal dilution. Hyoscyamus is a remedy that is called for when there is a lower grade of maniacal excitement than that which calls for Belladonna.*

*The Hyoscyamus patient is very exuberant in his expressions, but less frenzied than the Belladonna case. Hyoscyamus is very talkative, mostly good-natured and jolly. Occasionally he has savage outbursts, and is inclined to be destructive of clothing. The Hyoscyamus patient exposes the person because of lecherous thoughts and obscene tendencies. In this respect Hyoscyamus differs from Belladonna. As I have said, Belladonna tears off clothing for destructiveness; Hyoscyamus tears off clothing for the purpose of exposing the person, and for the purpose of exciting the passions of others. The Hyoscyamus patient is jolly and inclined to talk very much, and for this reason it is a suitable remedy for young, hysterical, nervous, and easily excited women.*

*The Stramonium patient unites some of the characteristics of Belladonna, Hyoscyamus, and Veratrum album. The Stramonium case is even more fierce than the Belladonna case. He has laughing fits like Hyoscyamus, or rather like a hyena; he waxes eloquent and pathetic in his despairings of salvation like the prover of Veratrum album; and he is also greatly troubled with hallucinations. Everything seems to be dark before his eyes. He swears at and makes threats against imaginary foes. He has periods when he is ready and "spoiling for a fight." But for the most part, the Stramonium case is an arrant and crouching coward. He sees animals, of strange varieties and gigantic proportions, leaping at him from the floor or the side walls, and he is greatly terrified by these apparitions.*

*Now remember this group of facts: Belladonna is fierce and brave; Hyoscyamus is jolly and companionable; Stramonium is wild and cowardly; Veratrum album is hopeless and despairing, or wildly plaintive, and beseeching for his salvation, which is apparently lost. Veratrum album is a remedy whose sphere of usefulness comprehends both profound prostration of the physical forces, and a most shattered condition of the intellectual faculties.*

*The fame of this drug extends over a period of more than three thousand years. It is related that about the year 1500 before the Christian Era, a certain Melampus, a celebrated physician among the Argives, is said to have cured the daughters of Proteus, King of the Argives, who, in consequence of remaining unmarried, were seized with an "amorous furor" and affected by a "wandering mania." These women had what is now called "old maid's insanity." They were cured chiefly by means of Veratrum album given in the milk of goats which had been fed upon that plant. We have verified the use of Veratrum album in "wandering mania," especially when the symptoms of peculiar excitement and tendency to travel are accompanied by great mental distress and physical collapse.*

*The Veratrum album patient combines, as primary effects, the wildest vagaries of the religious enthusiast, the amorous frenzies of the nymphomaniac, and the execrative passions of the infuriated demon, each striving for the ascendency, and causing the unfortunate victim to writhe and struggle with his mental and physical agonies, even as the dying Laocoön wrestled with the serpents of Minerva.*

*This anguish is short-lived. The patient soon passes from an exalted and frenzied condition into one of profound melancholia—abject despair of salvation, imbecile taciturnity, and complete prostration of both body and mind. The extremities become cold and blue, the heart's action is weak and irregular, the respiration is hurried, and all the objective symptoms are those of utter collapse. The physical state is like that of a case of cholera. At the same time the mind passes into a stygian gloom from which it slowly, if ever, emerges. With such a picture before us we can scarcely hesitate in the choice of a remedy, and Veratrum album is the one to be selected. There are, of course, cases which are past the grace of medicine, yet the earnest use of this long-tried drug has frequently repaid us by marked improvement following its administration, and in some cases Veratrum album has seemed to complete the cure.*

*We have portrayed a few characteristic symptoms of four drugs for the cure of insanity of the maniacal form. We might add to the list Aconite, with its high fever, its mental anxiety, its restlessness and fear of death. We might also speak of Veratrum viride, which has likewise an exalted temperature, a rapid pulse.*

*When there is great sexual excitement in mania, it may be relieved by the use of Cantharis. The Cantharis patient has frenzied paroxysms of an exalted type like Belladonna. The victim of this remedy bites and screams and tears his hair, and howls like a dog. As an invariable accompaniment, there is also great excitement of the sexual organism. In this latter respect Cantharis resembles Hyoscyamus and Veratrum album, but these latter drugs commingle the psychical with the physical, the Hyoscyamus patient displaying lively fancies in connection with erotic desires, and the Veratrum album patient uniting religious sentiment with lustful tendencies; but the Cantharis patient, on the other hand, is strictly and solely the embodiment of lechery for lechery's sake. This is a result of an intense erethism and inflammation of the sexual organs, impelling the victim to seek immediate physical gratification.*

*Again, we might speak of Nux vomica, which is a valuable remedy in subacute mania, where the patient is suspicious, and indulges in delusions of persecution and wrong. The Nux vomica patient is obstinate, incorrigible, cross, ugly, and sometimes studious. Bryonia is also an ugly remedy. The Nux vomica patient moves about, while the Bryonia patient keeps still because all his symptoms are aggravated by motion. [Note: recall Hans Burch Gram's report of a Nux vomica cure earlier.]*

We might also speak of Lachesis, which is a remedy for those who are extremely sensitive and persistently loquacious, and who indulge in the strange and fantastic idea that they are dead, and that preparations for the funeral are going on. The prover of Lachesis feels as if death had overtaken him, because of the profound and depressing effects of that powerful drug. The blood rot of Lachesis is only outrivaled by the blood rot of Baptisia tinctoria. The victim of the latter thinks that he is all to pieces and scattered about, while Lachesis only thinks that he is dead, and gathered to his fathers.

Rhus toxichodendron is of service in acute mania when there is a rheumatic history, an excessive restlessness at night, and when the patient is possessed of strong delusions of being poisoned. (Also Hyoscyamus and Veratrum viride.)

Tarantula is a remedy for crafty, cunning maniacs—patients who are full of mischief and prone to sudden fits of destructiveness, such as knocking down pictures, or sweeping bric-a-brac from a mantelpiece, or pounding a piano, or a helpless child.

Sulphur is useful in mania as an intercurrent remedy. Also for "fantastic mania" when the patient decks himself with gaudy colors, and puts on old rags of bright hues, and fancies them the most elegant decorations. Sulphur seldom achieves a cure by itself, but sometimes it seconds with vigor the efforts of other drugs.

## Paresis

For the relief of general paresis, we may suggest Mercury in its various forms, Nitric acid, Iodide of potash, Sulphur and Aurum if syphilis is suspected; and for the relief of the epileptiform seizures, Veratrum viride, Cimicifuga, Cuprum metallicum, and Laurocerasus. For the intense restlessness, anxiety, and expansive ideas, together with rapid emaciation of strength and flesh, you may use, according to the symptoms, Aconite, Arsenicum, Belladonna, and Cuprum. Alcohol produces artificial and temporary paresis, and is therefore homeopathic to the general article. It may be administered in small doses sometimes with benefit. Good whiskey, in one-half ounce doses, may be given once in three hours when necessary. The remedies have thus far not proven curative, but have sorry times afforded relief, and have seemed to affect a prolongation of life, and an increased comfort to the sick one.

## Dementia

Cases of dementia may require Anacardium if the patients are inclined to swear; Apium virus if the skin is puffy and smooth, and when there is inactivity of the kidneys; Calcarea carbonica when patients are fat, flabby and pale; Calcarea phosphoricum if there seems to be a tendency to cerebral chilblain; and Phosphoric acid when the patients are dull and drowsy with occasional periods of excitement, and profuse discharge of urine. In cases of profound mental depression and mental obfuscation—conditions which suggest both melancholia and dementia—when the nervous system is greatly exhausted, and when there are hysterical tendencies, and when the flow of urine is very profuse, Phosphoric acid is a leading remedy.

In masturbatic dementia we give Agnus castus, Causticum, Cantharis, Damiana, Picric acid, Phosphorus, Phosphoric acid, Staphisagria, Nux vomica, and Opium.

## Epilepsy

In epileptic dementia we sometimes find Belladonna, Cuprum aceticum, Laurocerasus, Enanthe crocata, and Solanum carolinense of service in relieving unfortunate symptoms. Enanthe crocata has done much good in the relief of epileptic insanity. Solanum carolinense has been used, but its effects seem to be cumulative, and while the fits may be checked for a season, they return with renewed vigor, and in a dangerous way.

Silicea, thirtieth, has been one of the most satisfactory remedies in effecting a wholesome change throughout the general physical system of the patient. As a health-developer in epilepsy, Silicea ranks as one of the first remedies on the list. In medicating epileptics, you should be careful and not overdo the work, and refrain from giving too much medicine. You should regulate the life, the diet, and the exposure to heat and wind. You should encourage the individual to a philosophical and natural state of living. You should provide against the injury of the patient during fits by covering everything that is hard, and by lining and padding everything which he is likely to strike. All sharp corners should be removed or covered in the room where the epileptic lives. His diet should be plain, wholesome, light, and not stimulating. If you give large doses of medicine and subdue or conceal the fits for a time, you subsequently find that you have simply postponed the evil day. You have worked cumulative *damage to your patient, and you have perhaps driven an otherwise quiet and harmless case into the toils of maniacal excitement, or into the deepest and most damnable depths of dementia.*

*For the relief of the epileptiform seizures, Veratrum viride, Cimicifuga, Cuprum metallicum, and Laurocerasus. For the intense restlessness, anxiety, and expansive ideas, together with rapid emaciation of strength and flesh, you may use, according to the symptoms, Aconite, Arsenicum, Belladonna, and Cuprum. Alcohol produces artificial and temporary paresis, and is therefore homeopathic to the genuine article. It may be administered in small doses, sometimes with benefit. Good whiskey, in one-half ounce doses, may be given once in three or four hours when necessary. These remedies have thus far not proved curative, but have sometimes afforded relief, and have seemed to effect a prolongation of life and an increased comfort to the sick one.*

## A SAMPLING OF CASE RECORDS

As privacy protections did not go into effect until 2003, case histories from bygone eras (with patient names deleted) are available for our perusal. The following are illustrative of Middletown Hospital care prior to 1900. The records appear in the *Twenty-Fourth Annual Report* on pages 99 to 131.

### *Case Summary One*

An 1875 Middletown Hospital case involving a pauperized twenty-five-year-old Irish Catholic housemaid suffering from maniacal attacks.

*Patient is naturally amiable and cheerful; about a year ago became homesick and nervous, and returned to Ireland; remained only a short time, and is said to have there shown some signs of insanity. About two weeks before her admission, was thrown from a wagon and hurt her head. A few days after, became depressed about the pecuniary and general welfare of her brother, whom she had, a short time before, induced to come to America. From this time her symptoms continued to increase in severity until she was brought to the asylum.*

## Treatment

*As of August 29, 1875, admission. Brought in last evening, about six o'clock, in a quiet state; at night insisted that she was dying and wanted a candle; went to sleep early, and slept until about eleven, P.M., then awoke in a phrensy of fright and rage; was sleeved, but tore them off and continued noisy until near morning; then slept about two hours; ate a good breakfast; pulse one hundred, and strong; tongue dry; pupils contracted; says she has been very thirsty; Acon [Aconite]. In afternoon fell asleep, but awoke at three; and at nine o'clock in same sort of rage as last night; Bell [Belladonna] to be given at time of the paroxysms. 8/30 slept well, pulse one hundred and four; appetite good; looks better. 8/31, slept well last night, and two hours to-day; pulse one hundred, and good; quieter; not excited; last night head less hot; tongue dry; very thirsty in the morning; says her head does not ache; Acon.*

*Sept. 2d. Excited yesterday; jacketed; slept well; inclined to be irritable; pulse less rapid; eats poorly; talks much about her brothers and her family. Sept. 3d. Slept well; excited at times; stamps around; seems to have some religious delusions; pulse 120; talks to herself. Sept. 4th, slept well, but ugly this morning; attacked every one she met; tried to bite; sleeved; Bell Sept. 5th. Commenced to flow very profusely last night; flow, bright red; Nux vom [vomica]. Sept. 6th. slept well; flowing less; Nux vom. Sept. 9th menses have ceased; pain in back part of head; slept poorly; Cimicifuga 30 C. Sept. 11th, less excited; pulse weak; sleeps and feels better; China. Sept. 15th mind much better; says she is only weak, and sometimes gets afraid. Sept. 20th, seems nearly well; stronger; pulse nearly normal; talks rationally; no excited paroxysms for some time; still has a burning sensation of the head; China. 9/22. Had a visit from her brother yesterday and is no worse for it; pulse better. Sept. 24th daily graining strength; had sore in occipital region; Arn [Arnica]. Sep. 25th quiet; complains still of soreness in occiput; sent to first ward; Arn. Oct. 10th. Discharged cured.*

The 1895 annual report of the Middletown State Homeopathic Hospital provides us with superintendent Dr. Maurice C. Ashley's "Synopsis of Twenty-One Critical Cases, and Some of the Special Features of Treatment of the Same at the Middletown State Homeopathic Hospital." By way of introduction Dr. Ashley says:

*During the past fifty years great strides have been made in the care and treatment of the insane. Liberal sums of money have been appropriated to build hospitals; physicians with ripened experience have been placed at the head of these institutions; men and women have been trained until they have become skillful nurses; chains and cruelty have been superseded by sympathetic and intelligent care, and food and medicines are carefully selected for each individual case. In fact, the "Bedlam" of but a comparatively few years since has given place to the most perfect system of caring for the insane that the world has ever known. The hospitals are large, comfortable and as homelike as is possible to make them, and they stand out boldly in every civilized country in the world as a glorious tribute to the charity of man to his fellow beings, and the advancement of mental science. Below I have endeavored to give a brief synopsis of twenty-one recent critical cases of insanity which have been cured at this hospital, together with some of the special features of the treatment applied.*

## Case Summary 2

*Female; admitted October 3, 1892; age, 45; single; American; seamstress; Protestant; education, academic; temperate; physical condition, weak; temperature, ninety-nine; on the pulse, 96; weight, eighty-six pounds; second attack; duration present attack, three months; exciting cause, physical disease. History previous to admission: Has attempted suicide; excited and depressed; violent but not dangerous; noisy; refuses to answer any questions whatever; pretends to be in prayer; calls on God to do various things; prayed and screamed loudly, and then lapsed into a quiet state with folded hands, devotional attitude; would answer no questions, but simply motion that she did not want to be disturbed; screamed, prayed and yelled night after night.*

*On admission was extremely restless; kept moving hands and feet constantly; appetite very poor. October eighth, severe diarrhoea set in, which lasted two months, reducing patient to almost a skeleton. October tenth, much quieter, sleeps better. Fifteenth, not eating or sleeping well. Twenty-fifth, writes poetry a great deal of the time, maniacal and incoherent. November tenth, weak and stupid; sleeps but little; restless at night. Fourteenth, excited, mouth dry and talks incoherently and constantly. November twenty-eighth, eating better, sleeps but little. December thirteenth, talking all the time, incoherent. Seventeenth, very excited and noisy. Twenty-third, still maniacal. Twenty-eighth, noisy and restless and disposed to be violent.*

*January 1, 1893, very noisy, awake all night. Third, delusions of poison, thinks the nurse is going to murder her, is very noisy, sleeps but little. January ninth, still noisy. From that time to February twenty-eighth not much change—excited, noisy, violent, indecent and obscene. At the end of this time she began to improve. March eighth, brighter; asks what month and day it is; realizes that she has been very ill; gaining in flesh; eating and sleeping better. April twelfth, much improved; has shown no mental aberrations for two weeks. May, patient still improving; continued to improve mentally and physically until September 26, 1893, at which time she was discharged recovered. Weight, 127 pounds, having gained forty-one pounds. Diagnosis, acute mania. Remedies—Hyos. [Hyoscyamus]; Bell. [Belladonna]; Arsen [Arsenis]; Aloes; l'odo.; Verat. Alb. [Veratrum album]; Sulph.[Sulphur]; Gels [Gelsemium]; Sepia.*

The spiritual frenzy she presents, not atypical of many cases, reflects the religiosity of the time as well as, I believe, a reverberation of post–Civil War grief and anguish.

------------------------

# The 1916 General Summary of Homeopathic Hospitals and Sanatoriums

With a view to standardizing and upgrading the quality of homeopathic education and homeopathic care, the American Institute of Homeopathy's Council on Medical Education prepared a report surveying and photographing hundreds of homeopathic asylums, hospitals, and homes. Though the oversight goal proved overly ambitious, a marvelous record of institutions under homeopathic management nevertheless emerged.[1]

Because policies keep evolving with changes in management and laws, as well as popular trends, it is not possible to definitively sort out the hospitals and sanatoriums specifically dedicated to the treatment of mental illness. However, we can present an accurate picture of homeopathic statistics in the early twentieth century.

- There are 101 institutions in the accredited class. These represent 20,092 beds.
- During the most recent reported upon fiscal years 109,527 hospital patients were treated.
- The average mortality rate in these institutions is 4.1 percent.
- There are required annually 248 interns to properly house-staff these hospitals.

- The estimated valuation of the properties of these strictly homeo-pathic institutions is $36,819,452.
- There are nineteen institutions in the registered class.
- There are here recorded 153 institutions that encourage and permit homeopathic physicians and treatment to be employed therein, with a strong probability that this number is greatly underestimated.
- In the Out-Door or Dispensary Departments of these institutions and those reporting to the Council, there were treated during the last fiscal year 287,887 patients.
- Allowing the same average number of patients for the nineteen registered hospitals as in the 101 in the accredited class, and counting dispensary cases, it is at once seen that during the past year there were treated in the charitable institutions of the Homeopathic School [meaning rendered homeopathic care] in the United States a total of 415,000 sick and injured persons.
- Add the number of patients treated homeopathically in the 153 institutions having homeopathic affiliation and we would have an approach to 750,000 of the hospital cases in the United States receiving annually therein homeopathic treatment.
- In states where a survey has been made indicating the medical faith of the population, it was found that actually 35.5 percent employ homeopathic treatment and 48.5 percent are kindly disposed toward homeopathy.
- In the training school for nurses connected with the purely homeopathic institutions there are enrolled 1,849 pupils.

# Resources

Links provided here offer additional information related to the contents of this book.

## ASYLUMS

**AsylumProjects.org.** Includes pages on the Cincinnati Sanitarium, the Gowanda State Hospital, and the Hudson River State Hospital.

**Substreet.org.** Website dedicated to stories and photographs of old sites, including several asylums discussed in this book.

## HOMEOPATHY

**GreenHealing.life.** Burke Lennihan's website offers books, blogs, and videos on natural healing.

**Homeoint.org.** Website for an international association of homeopaths, suppliers, educators, and individuals whose health has been improved by the use of homeopathic remedies. Membership fee supports the community and its informative website.

**Homeopathic.com.** Dana Ullman's long-running website offers books, courses, medicines, audio-video material, and commentary.

**Homeopathyusa.org.** Website for the American Institute of Homeopathy (AIH). Established in 1844, AIH is the oldest national medical association in the United States. Though members must belong to the medical community, the website's offerings of information on scientific developments relating to homeopathy are available for all.

**Hpathy.com.** Alan Schmukler's vibrant online journal and forum for homeopathy.

**Nature-reveals.com** (also known as Emryss). Website for Dutch publishing house offering state-of-the-art homeopathy and alternative and complementary medicine books.

**WholeHealthNow.com.** Kim Elia's comprehensive website offers software, an events calendar, and up-to-date information about homeopathy.

## LINCOLN

**AbrahamLincolnOnline.org.** A vast resource for books, educational courses, speeches, timeline, and scholarly developments regarding Abraham Lincoln.

**BataviaHistoricalSociety.org.** Batavia Depot Museum site. A portion of the site relates to Mary Todd Lincoln and includes archives, books, and photographs that record the history of the city and its families.

**FirstLadies.org.** The National First Ladies' Library features a useful bibliography of Mary Lincoln.

**KaneCountryConnects.com.** If you use the Search bar on this site to search on Mary Todd Lincoln, you'll find photographs and memorabilia about her stay in Batavia.

**Lincolncollection.tumblr.com.** Collection of Lincolniana and related materials including thousands of objects, nineteenth-century photographs, books, documents, and art related to Abraham Lincoln and his times.

**RogerjNorton.com.** Includes a Mary Todd Lincoln research site.

# Notes

PREFACE

1. Szasz, "Myth of Mental Illness," 116.
2. For instance, see the Middletown State Homeopathic Hospital page on photographer Tom Kirsch's website, Opacity.

INTRODUCTION. THE DEAD SEA SCROLLS
OF HOMEOPATHY AND PSYCHIATRY

1. Full Measure Staff, "The Dark Side of Wikipedia," Full Measure News (website), August 21, 2016.
2. Dale Steinreich, "100 Years of Medical Robbery," *Mises Daily Articles* (online), June 10, 2004.
3. Coulter, *Science and Ethics,* 120.
4. King, *History of Homeopathy,* vol. II, 14.
5. Winston, "Influenza–1918."
6. Whitaker, *Anatomy of an Epidemic,* 49–54.
7. Allsopp, Read, Corcoran, and Kinderman, "Heterogeneity in Psychiatric Diagnostic Classification," 15–22.

CHAPTER 1. WHO ARE THE MAD AND
WHERE SHALL THEY DWELL?

1. Szasz, "The Sane Slave," 333.
2. Szasz, "Myth of Mental Illness," 113.
3. Mayo Clinic Staff, "Anxiety Disorders," MayoClinic.org, accessed Nov. 2, 2021.
4. Mayo Clinic Staff, "PET scan of the brain for depression," MayoClinic.org, accessed Nov. 21, 2021.
5. Mayo Clinic Staff, "Epilepsy," MayoClinic (website), accessed Nov. 2, 2021.
6. Szasz, "Myth of Mental Illness," 115.
7. Szasz, "Myth of Mental Illness," 115.

8. Szasz, "Protocols of the Learned Experts on Heroin," 14, 20.

## CHAPTER 2. THE DAWN OF ENLIGHTENED MENTAL HEALTH CARE

1. Moylan and Baccolini, eds., *Utopia Method Vision*.
2. Geddes, Andreasen, and Goodwin, eds., *New Oxford Textbook of Psychiatry*, 23.
3. Sharfstein, "Madness, Morality, and Medicine."
4. "Thomas Story Kirkbride: The Story of the Magic Lantern," History of Pennsylvania Hospital, Stories, upenn.edu.
5. "Dr. Thomas Story Kirkbride," History of Pennsylvania Hospital, Historical Timeline, upenn.edu.
6. Goldstein and Godemont, "The Legend and Lessons of Geel."

## CHAPTER 3. HOMEOPATHY TO THE FORE

1. Robert Jütte, personal correspondence; see also Jütte, *Samuel Hahnemann*.
2. Robert Jütte, personal correspondence; see also Jütte, *Samuel Hahnemann*.
3. Sue Young Histories, "John Ernst Stapf 1788–1860," August 29, 2008.
4. Sylvain Cazalet, "American Homeopathy Was Started in Bath," Homéopathe International (website), 2003.
5. *WholeHealthNow* biography database, "Hans Burch Gram, M.D.," 2021.
6. Bradford, *Pioneers of Homeopathy*, 292.
7. Bradford, *Pioneers of Homeopathy*, 292–93.
8. Boger, *Boenninghausen's Characteristics Repertory*, s.v. "Nux vomica."

## CHAPTER 4. THE MADNESS OF MARY TODD LINCOLN

1. Spiegel and Kavaler, "The Role of Abraham Lincoln," abstract.
2. Hayden, *Pox*, 60.
3. Long, "Letters Shed New Light."
4. Sue Young Histories, "Tullio Suzzara Verdi 1829–1902," March 23, 2008.
5. Hayden, *Pox*, 128–29.
6. Rosenhek, "The First Lady of Lunacy."
7. Lincoln Collection, "'A Sad Revelation.'"
8. Abraham Lincoln Online, "Mary Lincoln at Bellevue Place."
9. Abraham Lincoln Online, "Mary Lincoln at Bellevue Place."
10. Abraham Lincoln Online, "Mary Lincoln at Bellevue Place."
11. Fairchild, *History of Medicine in Iowa*.
12. David Dyce Brown, *Permeation of Present Day Medicine by Homoeopathy*.

13. Brown, *Permeation of Present Day Medicine by Homoeopathy,* 1.
14. Dr. Kent Spender of Bath, "Notes on the Action of Medicines, New and Old," *British Medical Journal,* June 15, 1872.

## CHAPTER 5. ENTER SELDEN HAINES TALCOTT

1. Aldrich, "New York Homoepathic Medical College."
2. Talcott, *Hahnemann and His Influence.*
3. Whitaker, *Mad in America,* 34.
4. Mills, "History of the First Twenty-Five Years," 23.
5. Mills, "History of the First Twenty-Five Years," 23–26.
6. Mills, "History of the First Twenty-Five Years," 27–28.
7. Mills, "History of the First Twenty-Five Years," 28–29.
8. Mills, "History of the First Twenty-Five Years," 30.
9. O'Brien, "The Time When Americans Drank."
10. Sante, *Low Life,* 104.
11. Sante, *Low Life,* 105.
12. Cazalet, "History of Homoeopathy Biographies: Lilienthal, Samuel."
13. Lilienthal, *Homœopathic Therapeutics,* 253–54.
14. Sharma, "Dr. C. M. F. von Boenninghausen's Recommendations."
15. Talcott, *Hahnemann and His Influence.*
16. Ellis, *The Biography of John Stanton Gould.*
17. Wikipedia, "Middletown State Hospital," last edited on September 11, 2021.
18. Treuherz and Cazalet, *Homeopathic Hospitals and Sanatoriums.*
19. Talcott, *Mental Diseases and Their Modern Treatment,* "Hospital Construction" section following Lecture X (pages unnumbered).
20. Talcott, *Mental Diseases and Their Modern Treatment.*
21. Hughes, *Hudson Valley Psychiatric Hospitals.*
22. Davidson, *Century of Homeopaths,* 69.
23. Davidson, *Century of Homeopaths,* 69–70.
24. Talcott, "Freedom in Medical Matters."
25. American Medico-Psychological Association, *Proceedings* (1902), 324.

## CHAPTER 6. MIDDLETOWN STATE HOMEOPATHIC HOSPITAL'S UTOPIAN AGENDA

1. Asylum Projects (website), s.v. "Middletown State Hospital."
2. Whitaker, *Mad in America,* 34.
3. Leclercq, "American Homeopathic Psychiatry."
4. State of New York, *State Commission in Lunacy,* 104.
5. Middletown State Homoeopathic Hospital, *Twenty-Fourth Annual Report,* 24.

6. Dwyer, *Homes for the Mad,* 52; Grob, *The State and the Mentally Ill,* 163, 226–27.
7. Samuel Worcester, untitled, Transactions of the HMSSNY, Proceedings of the 21st Annual Meeting 10 (1872):15–6., 22 Ibid., 16–7.
8. Leclercq, "American Homeopathic Psychiatry."

## CHAPTER 7. WALKING THE TALK

1. Middletown State Homoeopathic Hospital, *Twelfth Annual Report,* 21.
2. Middletown State Homoeopathic Hospital, *Twelfth Annual Report,* 21, cited by Panciroli.
3. Talcott, *Mental Diseases and Their Modern Treatment.*
4. Asylum Projects (website), s.v. "Hudson River State Hospital."
5. Galante, *Images of America,* 65.
6. Croyle, "Inside 'Old Main.'"
7. Clark, *A Century of Progress,* 7–12.
8. Smith, "Lunatic Asylum in the Workhouse."

## CHAPTER 8. PLAY BALL!
## THE INNOVATION OF BASEBALL THERAPY

1. "The Diamond Way: Baseball as an Esoteric Ritual," written and illustrated by Hannah M. G. Shapero and originally published in *Gnosis* magazine."
2. Kawakami et al., "Influence of Watching Professional Baseball."

## CHAPTER 9. GENIUS PHYSICIAN AND
## NURSE-EDUCATOR CLARA BARRUS

1. Cazalet, "History of the New York Medical College and Hospital for Women."
2. Masiello, "Homeopathy."
3. Anthony, *Selected Papers.*
4. Obituary of Susan Ann Edson, *The Moulton Advertiser,* November 18, 1897, p. 1.

## CHAPTER 10. DISCIPLES AND SATELLITES
## OF THE MOTHER CHURCH

1. Talcott, "New Methods."
2. Holtzman, "A Home Away from Home."
3. "Westborough State Hospital," Opacity (website).
4. "Westborough State Hospital," Opacity (website).
5. Westborough Hospital Annual Reports.
6. Butler Hospital, *Butler Hospital,* 8.

7. Butler Hospital, *Butler Hospital,* 19.

8. Butler Hospital, *Butler Hospital,* 22.

9. Butler Hospital, *Butler Hospital,* 16–18.

10. Sue Young Histories, "The Wesselhoeft Family and Homeopathy," December 20, 2007.

11. Cleave, *Cleave's Biographical Cyclopædia.*

12. Davidson, *Century of Homeopaths,* 69.

13. Worcester, *Insanity and Its Treatment,* 149–51.

14. Worcester, *Insanity and Its Treatment,* 384–85.

15. Asylum Projects (website), s.v. "Gowanda Homeopathic State Hospital."

16. Asylum Projects (website), s.v. "Cincinnati Sanitarium."

17. Everett, *Biological History of Eminent and Self-Made Men.*

18. Sundquist-Nassie, "I Wish You Abundant Reward."

19. Asylum Projects (website), s.v. "The Easton Sanitarium."

20. "Dr. Amos Jay Givens," Find a Grave (website), January 4, 2016.

21. Stamford Advocate, Obituary.

22. Stamford Advocate, Obituary.

23. Stamford Advocate, Obituary.

24. Givens, Amos, in *Pamphlets-Homoeopathic: Nervous Diseases,* volume 2, page 20.

25. Substreet: History Under Ground (website), s.v. "Fergus Falls State Hospital."

26. Davidson, *Century of Homeopaths,* 76.

## CHAPTER II. CONCESSIONS TO THE SPIRIT OF THE TIMES

1. Friedman, "Menninger."

2. My clinical experience with this point is reported in the article "Been Diagnosed with Cancer or Know Someone Who Has? Talk to Your Acupuncturist about the 'Root of Tumor' Acupoint," Vital Force Health Care website, December 10, 2015.

3. López-Muñoz, "History of the Discovery."

4. E. Richard Brown, "Rockefeller Medicine Men."

5. "Butler, William Morris" in King, *History of Homeopathy.*

6. Butler, *Mental Diseases,* preface.

7. Rayner, "75 Years of Help."

8. Klopp, Initial Superintendent's Report dated 1912–1914, cited by Rayner, "75 Years of Help."

9. Davidson, *Century of Homeopaths,* 76.

10. Rayner, "75 Years of Help."

11. Rayner, "75 Years of Help."
12. Rayner, "75 Years of Help."
13. Davidson, *Century of Homeopaths,* 74–75.
14. Rayner, "75 Years of Help."
15. Davidson, *Century of Homeopaths,* 76.
16. Kansas Historical Society, "Papers of Charles Frederick Menninger."
17. Kansas Historical Society, "Menninger Clinic."
18. Davidson, *Century of Homeopaths,* 81.
19. Davidson, *Century of Homeopaths,* 77.
20. Davidson, *Century of Homeopaths,* 84.
21. Davidson, *Century of Homeopaths,* 76.
22. "A History of the Fergus Falls Treatment Center," July 16, 2004, Minnesota Public Radio News and Features.
23. Davidson, *Century of Homeopaths,* 77.
24. Davidson, *Century of Homeopaths,* 77.
25. Davidson, *Century of Homeopaths,* 72–73.
26. *New York Times* staff, "Dr. Winfred Overholser Dies."
27. Arnold & Porter, "Insanity and the Law."
28. Edric Lescouflair. "Overholser, Winfred (1892–1964): Biographical Introduction." Harvard Square Library (website). Accessed November 5, 2021.

## CHAPTER 12. INVESTING IN SANITY

1. Granger, "Discovery of Haloperidol."
2. "Haloperidol: Drug Usage Statistics, United States, 2013–2019," ClinCalc .com.
3. Whitaker, *Anatomy of an Epidemic,* 267.
4. Julian, *Materia Medica of New Homoeopathic Remedies.*
5. Chase, *Harvard and the Unabomber.*
6. Kresser, "The 'Chemical Imbalance' Myth."
7. Kresser, "The 'Chemical Imbalance' Myth."
8. Malin, and Saleh, "Paraphilias."

## APPENDIX 1. COMPENDIUM OF MADNESS PERSPECTIVES

1. Whitaker, "Polypharmacy/Bipolar Disorder."
2. Payne, *Confessions of a Taoist on Wall Street,* 153.
3. Chen, "Articulating 'Chinese Madness."
4. A classification from Edmund Burke Huey, *Backward and Feeble-Minded Children* (1912).

5. Foucault, *Madness and Civilization.*

6. Robbins, *Cezanne in Britain.*

7. Kantor, "Cyclical Remedy Complexes."

8. Reich, *Mass Psychology of Fascism,* 192.

9. Firstenberg, *Invisible Rainbow,* 50–65 and throughout the work.

10. Marland, *Dangerous Motherhood,* 135.

11. Marks, "Book review of *Dangerous Motherhood.*"

12. Askovic et al., "Evaluation of Neurofeedback for Posttraumatic Stress Disorder."

13. Caldwell and Van Rybroek, "Efficacy of a Decompression Treatment."

14. Kantor, *Interpreting Chronic Illness,* 99.

## APPENDIX 2. EXEMPLIFYING NANOMEDICINE: THE RESEARCH OF DR. IRIS BELL

1. Ellis, "Federal Jury Clears Producer."

2. Bell and Schwartz, "Adaptive Network Nanomedicine."

3. van der Post et al., "Strong Frequency Dependence."

4. Chirumbolo and Bjorklund. "Homeopathic Dilutions."

5. Rao, Roy, Bell, and Hoover. "The Defining Role of Structure."

6. Klotter, "New Science Supports Homeopathy."

7. Bell, Iris R., and Gary E. Schwartz. "Enhancement of Adaptive Biological Effects."

8. Walach, H. "Entanglement Model of Homeopathy as an Example."

9. Bell and Koithan. "A Model for Homeopathic Remedy Effects."

10. Zhang and An, "Cytokines, Inflammation and Pain."

11. Zhang and An, "Cytokines, Inflammation and Pain."

12. Zhang and An, "Cytokines, Inflammation and Pain."

13. Arora, "Dehydroepiandrosterone (DHEA)."

14. Pizzino et al., "Oxidative Stress."

15. Bell and Koithan, "A Model for Homeopathic Remedy Effects."

## APPENDIX 3. SAMUEL HAHNEMANN'S MENTAL HEALTH APHORISMS

1. International Academy of Classical Homeopathy (website), "Aphorisms 210–230."

## APPENDIX 5. THE 1916 GENERAL SUMMARY OF HOMEOPATHIC HOSPITALS AND SANATORIUMS

1. American Institute of Homeopathy, *Hospitals and Sanatoriums of the Homoeopathic School of Medicine.*

# Bibliography

Abraham Lincoln Online. "Mary Lincoln at Bellevue Place." Abraham Lincoln Online (website), 2019.

Aldrich, Henry C., ed. *Minneapolis Homoeopathic Magazine,* vol. 7, 1898.

Aldrich, L. C. "The New York Homoepathic Medical College and Hospital." Chapter IX in *History of Homoepathy and its Institutions in America* by William Harvey King, M. D., LL. D., presented by Sylvain Cazalet.

Allsopp, Kate, John Read, Rhiannon Corcoran, and Peter Kinderman. "Heterogeneity in Psychiatric Diagnostic Classification." *Psychiatry Research* 279 (2019): 15–22.

American Institute of Homeopathy, Council on Medical Education. *Hospitals and Sanatoriums of the Homoeopathic School of Medicine: With One Hundred and Ninety-Nine Illustrations in the Text.* American Institute of Homoeopathy, 1916.

American Medico-Psychological Association. Proceedings of the Annual Meeting. Utica, N.Y., 1894.

American Medico-Psychological Association. Proceedings of the Annual Meeting. Utica, N.Y., 1902.

American Psychiatric Association. *Diagnostic and Statistical Manual of Mental Disorders (DSM-5).* Washington, D.C.: American Psychiatric Association Publishing, 2013.

Anthony, Susan Brownell, et al. *The Selected Papers of Elizabeth Cady Stanton and Susan B. Anthony: In the School of Anti-slavery, 1840 to 1866.* New Brunswick, N.J.: Rutgers University Press, 1997.

Arnold, Thurman. "Insanity and the Law, Part I: The Strange Case of Ezra Pound." Arnold & Porter (website) News and Perspectives, 1996.

Arora, Puneet. "Dehydroepiandrosterone (DHEA)." Hormone Health Network (online). Last updated May 2019.

Askovic, M., A. J. Watters, M. Coello, J. Aroche, A. W. F. Harris, J. Kropotov. "Evaluation of Neurofeedback for Posttraumatic Stress Disorder Related to Refugee Experiences Using Self-Report and Cognitive ERP Measures." *Clinical EEG and Neuroscience.* 51, no. 2 (2020): 79–86.

Baker, Jean H. *Mary Todd Lincoln: A Biography*. New York: W. W. Norton & Co., 1989.

Banta, Richard Elwell, ed. *Indiana Authors and Their Books:* "Everts, Orpheus: 1826–1903." Crawfordsville, Ind.: Wabash College, 1949.

Barrus, Clara. *Nursing the Insane*. New York: Macmillan, 1915. A Scholar Select, Wentworth Press reprint.

———. *Whitman and Burroughs, Comrades*. Port Washington, N.Y.: Kennikat Press, 1968.

Bell, Iris R., and Mary Koithan. "A Model for Homeopathic Remedy Effects: Low Dose Nanoparticles, Allostatic Cross-Adaptation, and Time-Dependent Sensitization in a Complex Adaptive System." *BMC Complementary and Alternative Medicine* 12, no. 191 (October 2012).

Bell, Iris R., and Gary E. Schwartz. "Adaptive Network Nanomedicine: An Integrated Model for Homeopathic Medicine." *Frontiers in Bioscience (Scholar Edition)* 5, no. 2 (2013): 685–708.

———. "Enhancement of Adaptive Biological Effects by Nanotechnology Preparation Methods in Homeopathic Medicines." *Homeopathy* 104, no. 2 (2015): 123–38.

Blumer, G. Alder, M.D., et al. eds. *American Journal of Insanity,* vol. LXIV. Baltimore: The Johns Hopkins Press/The Lord Baltimore Press, July 1907, p. 64.

Boger, C. M. *Boenninghausen's Characteristics Repertory*. Clifton Park, N.Y.: Nanopathy, 2011.

Bradford, Thomas Lindsley. *The Pioneers of Homeopathy*. Philadelphia: Boericke & Tafel, 1897.

Brown, David Dyce. *The Permeation of Present Day Medicine by Homoeopathy*. London: Forgotten Books, 2019. Reprint authorized by the British Homeopathic Association. 1904. A Nabu Public Domain Reprint.

Brown, Norman O. *Life Against Death: The Psychoanalytical Meaning of History*. Middletown, Conn.: Wesleyan University Press, 1985.

———. *Loves Body*. Oakland: University of California Press, 1990.

Brown, E. Richard. *Rockefeller Medicine Men: Medicine and Capitalism in America*. Berkeley: University of California Press, 1979.

Butler, William Morris. *Mental Diseases and Their Homoeopathic Treatment: For the Student and Practitioner of Medicine*. New York: Boericke & Runyon, 1910. A University of Michigan Library digitization project reprint.

Butler Hospital. *The Butler Hospital: Its Story*. Providence, R.I.: Trustees and Superintendent of Butler Hospital, 1926.

Caldwell, Michael F., and Gregory J. Van Rybroek. "Efficacy of a Decompression

Treatment Model in the Clinical Management of Violent Juvenile Offenders." 45, no. 4 (2001).

Cazalet, Sylvain, presenter. "History of Homoeopathy Biographies: Butler, William Morris." Homéopathe International (website), 2003.

———, presenter. "History of the New York Medical College and Hospital for Women." Homéopathe International (website), 2001.

———, presenter. "History of Homoeopathy Biographies: Lilienthal, Samuel." Homéopathe International (website), 2002.

Chase, Alston. *Harvard and the Unabomber: The Education of an American Terrorist.* New York: W. W. Norton, 2003.

Chen, Hsiu-fen. "Articulating 'Chinese Madness': A Review of the Modern Historiography of Madness in Pre-Modern China." The First Annual Meeting, Academia Sinica. National Chengchi University: Department of History, November 4–8, 2003.

Chirumbolo, Salvatore, and Geir Bjorklund. "Homeopathic Dilutions, Hahnemann, and the Solvent Issue: Must We Address Ethanol as a 'Homeopathic' or a 'Chemical' Issue?" *Homeopathy* 107, no. 1 (February 2018): 40–44.

Clark, Lucy. "A Century of Progress at Utica State Hospital 1843–1943." Utica, N.Y.: Utica State Hospital Alumnae Association, 1943.

Cleave, Egbert. *Cleave's Biographical Cyclopaedia of Homeopathic Physicians and Surgeons.* Philadelphia: Galaxy, 1873.

Coulter, Harris L. *The Conflict between Homeopathy and the American Medical Association. Divided Legacy,* vol. 3. Wehawken, N.J.: Wehawken Book Company, 1973.

———. *A History of the Schism in Medical Thought. Divided Legacy,* vol. 4, Berkeley, Calif.: North Atlantic Books, 1982.

———. *Science and Ethics in American Medicine, 1800–1914.* Wehawken, N.J.: Wehawken Book Company, 1973.

Croyle, Jonathan. "Inside 'Old Main,' Utica's Psychiatric Hospital." Syracuse.com, CNY Vintage, May 19, 2016. Updated March 22, 2019.

Davidson, Jonathan. *A Century of Homeopaths: Their Influence on Medicine and Health.* New York: Springer, 2014.

De Young, Mary. *Encyclopedia of Asylum Therapeutics, 1750–1950s.* Jefferson, N.C.: McFarland & Company, Inc., 2015.

———. *Madness: An American History of Mental Illness and Its Treatment.* Jefferson, N.C.: McFarland & Company, Inc., 2010.

Dougherty, Edward P. "Centennial Chronicle: The Story of 100 Years of the Middletown State Hospital." Fourth Annual Report for the Year ending November 30, 1974. Middletown, N.Y.: Trumbull Printing, 1974.

Dwyer, Ellen. *Homes for the Mad: Life inside Two Nineteenth-Century*

*Asylums*. New Brunswick, N.J.: Rutgers University Press, 1987.

Ellis, Captain Franklin. *Biography of John Stanton Gould*. Philadelphia: Everts & Ensign, pp. 198–99.

Ellis, Tucker. "Federal Jury Clears Producer, Marketer, and Seller of Homeopathic Products in $255M Class Action Trial." Lexology (website). September 18, 2015.

Emerson, Jason. *Giant in the Shadows: The Life of Robert T. Lincoln*. Carbondale, Ill.: Southern Illinois University Press, 2012.

———. *The Madness of Mary Lincoln*. Carbondale, Ill.: Southern Illinois University Press, 2007.

*Encyclopedia of Mental Disorders*. Definition of Exhibitionism. Minddisorders .com.

Everett, Craig, interpreter. "A Biological History of Eminent and Self-Made Men of the State of Indiana." Cincinnati: Western Biographical Publishing Company, 1880.

Executive documents for the State of Minnesota, vol. III. St. Paul, Minn.: Pioneer Press Company, 1895.

Fairchild, D. S. *History of Medicine in Iowa*. Des Moines: Iowa State Medical Society, 1927.

Faust, Drew Gilpin. *The Republic of Suffering, Death, and the American Civil War*. New York: Vintage, 2008.

Fiesthumel, Scott. *"Pent-Ups": Minor League Baseball in Utica, New York 1878–1892*. Self-published history, 1995.

Finta, Susan. "Clara Barton, a Lifetime of Service." Clara Barton National Historic Site, a division of the National Park Service. Accessed December 3, 2021.

Firstenbirg, Arthur. *The Invisible Rainbow: A History of Electricity and Life*. Hartford, Vt.: Chelsea Green, 2017.

Foucault, Michel. Madness and Civilization: A History of Insanity in the Age of Reason. Translated by Richard Howard. New York: Vintage, 1988.

Friedman, Lawrence J. "Menninger, the Family and the Clinic." Review of *The Hospital the Menningers Built,* by Howard Markel. Washington Post website, September 18, 1990.

Galante, Joseph, Lynn Rightmyer, and the Hudson River State Hospital Nurses Alumni Association. *Images of America: Hudson River State Hospital*. Charleston, S.C.: Arcadia Publishing, 2018.

Gallavardin, Jean-Pierre. *The Homeopathic Treatment of Alcoholism,* Philadelphia: Hahnemann Publishing House, 1890.

Gardner, Dennis P. *Minnesota Treasures: Stories Behind the State's Historic Places*. St. Paul: Minnesota State Historical Society Press, 2004.

Geddes, John, Nancy C. Andreasen, and Guy M. Goodwin, ed. *New Oxford Textbook of Psychiatry*. Third edition. Oxford, U.K.: Oxford University Press, 2020.

Goldstein, Jackie L., and Marc M. L. Godemont. "The Legend and Lessons of Geel, Belgium: A 1500-Year-Old Legend, a 21st-Century Model." *Community Mental Health Journal* 39, no. 5 (2003): 441–58.

Granger, B. "The Discovery of Haloperidol." *Encephale* 25, no. 1 (Jan.–Feb. 1999): 59–66.

Grob, Gerald N. *The State and the Mentally Ill: A History of Worcester State Hospital in Massachusetts, 1830–1920*. Chapel Hill: University of North Carolina Press, 1966.

Haehl, Richard, M.D., and *The Lesser Writings of Samuel Hahnemann*. London: Andesite Press, 2017.

Haehl, Richard, M.D., and Marie L. Wheeler, trans. *Hahnemann, His Life and Work*. London: Homoeopathic Publishing Company, n.d. Digitized by the Internet Archive in 2017 (website).

Hahnemann, Samuel. *The Organon of Medicine, Fifth & Sixth Edition Combined*. Gazelle Distribution Trade, 2009.

Hayden, Deborah. *Pox: Genius, Madness, and the Mysteries of Syphilis*. New York: Basic Books, 2003.

Hirschhorn, Norbert, and Feldman, Robert G. "Mary Lincoln's Final Illness: A Medical and Historical Reappraisal." *Journal of the History of Medicine*, October 1999.

Holtzman, Ellen. "A Home away from Home: Luxurious Accommodations Were the Staples of America's Gilded Age Asylums, which Offered State-of-the-Science Treatment—for the Rich Only." *American Psychological Association* 43, no. 3 (March 2012): 24.

Hudson River State Hospital Annual Reports: United States, n.p, 1868. Asylum Projects (website).

Huey, Edmund Burke. *Backward and Feeble-Minded Children: Clinical Studies in the Psychology of Defectives, With a Syllabus for the Clinical Examination and Testing of Children*. Baltimore: Warwick and York, 1912.

Hughes, C. J. *Hudson Valley Psychiatric Hospitals: Insane Asylums and Psych Centers of Upstate New York*. Hudson Valley email newsletter, 9/13/2011.

Jansen, Ton, *Fighting Fire with Fire, Homeopathic Detox Therapy*. Sofia, Bulgaria: Anhira, Ltd., 2016.

Johnson, Emory, Jr., comp. *A Short History of the Fergus Falls State Hospital, Fergus Falls, Minnesota*, June 1972. Substreet (website).

Julian, A. O. *Materia Medica of New Homoeopathic Remedies*. Beaconsfield Publishers: Found in Reference Works homeopathic software under Haloperidol (non-paginated), 1984.

Jütte, Robert. *Samuel Hahnemann: The Founder of Homeopathy.* Translated from German by Margot Saar, 2012. Munich: dtv, 2005.

Kansas Historical Society. *Menninger Foundation Archives.* Created: December 2004, modified: July 2017.

Kantor, Jerry. *Autism Reversal Toolbox. Strategies, Remedies, Resources.* Haarlem, Netherlands: Emryss, 2015.

———. "Cyclical Remedy Complexes: Their Origin within Traditional Chinese Medicine and Relevance for Miasmatic Theory." *Homœopathic Links* 30, no. 3 (2017): 202–7.

———. *Interpreting Chronic Illness, the Convergence of Traditional Chinese Medicine, Homeopathy and Biomedicine.* Wellesley Hills, Mass.: Right Whale Press, 2011.

Karst, F. "Homeopathy in Illinois." *Caduceus: A Museum Quarterly for the Health Sciences* (Summer 1988): 1–33.

Kawakami, Ryoko, et al. "Influence of Watching Professional Baseball on Japanese Elders' Affect and Subjective Happiness." *Gerontology and Geriatric Medicine* 3 (2017).

King, William Harvey, ed. *History of Homeopathy and Its Institutions in America, vol. 3.* Whitefish, Mont.: Kessinger Publishing, 2010.

Kirsch, Tom *Crumbling Castles: The Lost Asylums at Worcester and Danvers.* Charleston, S.C.: America Through Time, October 28, 2019.

———. "Westborough State Hospital, an Abandoned Psychiatric Hospital." Opacity (website).

Kirschmann, Anne Taylor. *A Vital Force, Women in American Homeopathy.* New Brunswick, N.J.: Rutgers University Press, 2004.

Klotter, Julie. "New Science Supports Homeopathy." *Townsend Letter* (website). Accessed 10/25/21.

Kratzer, Al. *The Easton Sanitarium,* College Hill, Easton History. November 2, 2014. House on College Hill (website).

Kresser, Chris. "The 'Chemical Imbalance' Myth." *Chris Kresser* (fact-checked blog). Last updated June 19, 2019.

Laing, R. D. *The Divided Self.* London: Penguin Books, rev. ed., 1965.

Lansky, Amy. *Impossible Cure: the Promise of Homeopathy.* Portola Valley, Calif.: R. L. Ranch Press, 2003.

Leclercq, Valerie. "American Homeopathic Psychiatry and the Promise of Patient-Centered Asylum Care: The Middletown Homoeopathic State Hospital (1870–1910). Available at Academia (website).

Lescouflair, Edric. *Winfred Overholser, (1892–1964), Biographical Introduction.* Harvard Square Library website. Accessed Jan. 29, 2022.

Leskowitz, Eric, *The Joy of Sox: Weird Science and the Power of Intention.* North Charleston, S.C.: CreateSpace, 2010.

Lilienthal, Samuel. *Homœopathic Therapeutics.* Philadelphia: Hahnemann Publishing House, 1890.

Lincoln Collection. "'A Sad Revelation': The Insanity Trial of Mary Todd Lincoln." Lincoln Collection tumblr post (online), March 27, 2017.

Long, Ray. "Letters Shed New Light on Mary Lincoln's Thoughts." *Chicago Tribune,* September 9, 1999.

López-Muñoz, F., C. Alamo, E. Cuenca, W. Shen, P. Clervoy, and G. Rubio. "History of the Discovery and Clinical Introduction of Chlorpromazine" *Annals of Clinical Psychiatry* 17, no. 3 (2005): 113–35.

Malin, H. Martin, and Fabian M. Saleh. "Paraphilias: Clinical and Forensic Considerations." *Psychiatric Times* 24, no. 5 (Apr. 15, 2007), 32.

Marks, Lara. "Book Review: *Dangerous Motherhood: Insanity and Childbirth in Victorian Britain. Medical History* 50, no. 1 (2006): 135–36.

Marland, Hilary. *Dangerous Motherhood: Insanity and Childbirth in Victorian Britain.* New York: Palgrave Macmillan, 2004.

Masiello, Domenick. "Homeopathy." In *The Illustrated Encyclopedia of Body-Mind Disciplines,* edited by Nancy Allison. New York: Rosen Publishing, 1999.

Mayer, Bob. "The Asylum Base Ball Club, Middletown's Crack Semi-Pro Team 1888–94." Clifford Blau Original Baseball Research (website).

McCabe, Vinton. *Let Like Cure Like: The Definitive Guide to the Healing Powers of Homeopathy.* New York: St. Martin's Press, 1997.

Menninger, Charles Frederick. *Papers of Charles Frederick Menninger.* Kansas Historical Society, 1884–1969.

Middletown State Homoeopathic Hospital. *Twelfth Annual Report of the State Homoeopathic Asylum for the Insane at Middletown, N.Y.* Albany, N.Y.: Weed, Parsons and Company, 1883.

———. *Sixteenth Annual Report of the State Homoeopathic Asylum for the Insane.* Albany, N.Y.: The Argus Company, 1887.

———. *Twenty-Fourth Annual Report of the Middletown State Homeopathic Hospital at Middletown, N.Y.* Albany, N.Y.: James B. Lyon, State Printer, 1895.

Mills, Walter Sands. *History of the First Twenty-Five Years of the Ward's Island and Metropolitan Hospital, 1875–1900. Also an Account of Its Graduates.* New York: Rooney & Otten, 1900.

Minnesota Bureau of Labor Biennial Report, 1904.

Minnesota Federal Writers' Project. *Minnesota: A State Guide.* New York: Viking Press, 1938.

Minnesota Public Radio. *History of the Fergus Falls Treatment Center.* Collegeville, Minn.: News and Features, July 16, 2004.

Moulton Advertiser. Obituary: Dr. Susan A. Edson. Moulton, Ala., November 18, 1897.

Moylan, Thomas, and Raffaella Baccolini, eds. *Utopia Method Vision: The Use Value of Social Dreaming.* Bern, Switzerland: Peter Lang, 2007.

Neely, Mark E., Jr., and Gerald R. McMurtry. *The Insanity File: The Case of Mary Todd Lincoln.* Carbondale, Ill.: Southern Illinois University Press, 1993.

*New York Times* staff. "Dr. Winfred Overholser Dies." *Obituary,* October 7, 1964, pg. 47.

Noll, Richard. *American Madness: The Rise and Fall of Dementia Praecox.* Cambridge, Mass.: Harvard University Press, 2011

O'Brien, Jane. "The Time When Americans Drank All Day Long." *BBC News,* March 9, 2015.

Panciroli, Paola. "The Asylum as Utopia in the Homeopathic Landscape: Innovations and Contradictions." *Societate si Politica; Arad* 12, no. 1 (2018).

Payne, David. *Confessions of a Taoist on Wall Street.* Boston: Houghton Mifflin, 1984.

Photothèque Homéopathique. "Dr. Tullio Suzzara Verdi (1829–1902)." Homéopathe International, 2009.

Pizzino, G., N. Irrera, M. Cucinotta, G. Pallio, F. Mannino, V. Arcoraci, F. Squadrito, D. Altavilla, and A. Bitto. "Oxidative Stress: Harms and Benefits for Human Health." *Oxid Med Cell Longev* 2017 (2017).

Rao, Manju Lata, Rustum Roy, Iris R. Bell, and Richard Hoover. "The Defining Role of Structure (Including Epitaxy) in the Plausibility of Homeopathy." *Homeopathy* 96, no. 3 (2007): 175–82.

Rayner, Polly. "75 Years of Help, Healing Numerous Activities Will Note Allentown State Hospital's Gains." *The Morning Call,* October 4, 1987.

Reich, William. *The Mass Psychology of Fascism.* Vincent R. Carfagno, trans. New York: Farrar, Straus, & Giroux, 1970.

Robbins, Anne. *Cezanne in Britain.* London: National Gallery, 2006.

Robins, Natalie. *Copeland's Cure, Homeopathy and the War Between Conventional and Alternative Medicine.* New York: Knopf, 2005.

Rosenhek, Jackie. "The First Lady of Lunacy." Doctor's Review (website), November 3, 2021.

Ross, Rodney A. "Mary Todd Lincoln, Patient at Bellevue Place, Batavia." *Journal of the Illinois State Historical Society,* Spring 1970.

Sante, Luc. *Low Life, Lures, and Snares of Old New York.* New York: Random House Inc., 1992.

Shapero, Hannah M. G. "The Diamond Way: Baseball as an Esoteric Ritual." SouthernCrossReview (website). Accessed Nov. 5, 2021.

Sharfstein, Steven. "Madness, Morality and Medicine: A Study of the York Retreat, 1796–1914." *Journal of the American Medical Association.* 256, no. 7 (1986): 931.

Sharma, Saumya, "Dr. C.M.F. von Boenninghausen's Recommendations in Treating Alcohol Use Disorder." See Homeopathy Papers on Hpathy (website). May 18, 2019.

Smith, Leonard. "Lunatic Asylum in the Workhouse: St Peter's Hospital, Bristol, 1698–1861." *Medical History* 61, no. 2 (2017): 225–45.

Smits, Tinus. *Autism Beyond Despair, CEASE Therapy,* Emryss, 2010.

So, James Tin Yau. *The Book of Acupuncture Points (Complete Course in Acupuncture, vol 1).* Brookline, Mass.: Paradigm Publications, 1985.

Spiegel, Allen D., and Florence Kavaler. "The Role of Abraham Lincoln in Securing a Charter for a Homeopathic Medical College." Journal of Community Health 27, no. 5: 357–80.

Stamford Advocate. Obituary: Dr. Amos J. Givens. Stamford, Conn., July 8, 1919.

State of Minnesota. Legislative manual, 1907.

State of New York. *State Commission in Lunacy Seventh Annual Report, October 1, 1894, to September 30, 1895.* Albany and New York: Wynkoop Hallenbeck Craford, 1896.

Stuhler, Linda S. *The Inmates of Willard 1870 to 1900: A Genealogy Resource* (blog). Last updated November 7, 2020.

Sundquist-Nassie, Linda. "I Wish You Abundant Reward: The Life of Dr. Orpheus Everts, Surgeon—20th Indiana." National Museum of Civil War Medicine website, December 7th, 2014.

Szasz, Thomas. The Age of Madness: A History of Involuntary Mental Hospitalization Presented in Selected Texts (editor). London: Routledge & Kegan Paul Ltd., 1975 [1973].

———. *Coercion as Cure: A Critical History of Psychiatry.* New Brunswick, N.J.: Transaction Publishers, 2007.

———. *Cruel Compassion: Psychiatric Control of Society's Unwanted.* Syracuse N.Y.: Syracuse University Press, 1998 [1994].

———. *Heresies.* New York: Doubleday Anchor, 1976.

———. *Insanity: The Idea and Its Consequences.* Syracuse, N.Y.: Syracuse University Press, 1997 [1987].

———. *A Lexicon of Lunacy: Metaphoric Malady, Moral Responsibility, and Psychiatry.* New Brunswick, N.J.: Transaction Publishers, 2003 [1993].

———. *Liberation by Oppression: A Comparative Study of Slavery and Psychiatry.* New Brunswick, N.J.: Transaction Publishers, 2002.

———. *The Medicalization of Everyday Life: Selected Essays.* Syracuse, N.Y.: Syracuse University Press. 2007.

———. *The Myth of Mental Illness.* New York: Harper, 1961.

———. "The Myth of Mental Illness." *American Psychologist* 15 (1960): 113–18.

———. *The Myth of Psychotherapy: Mental Healing as Religion, Rhetoric, and Repression.* Syracuse, N.Y.: Syracuse University Press, 1988 [1978].

———. *Pharmacracy: Medicine and Politics in America.* Westport, Conn.: Praeger Publishers, 2001.

———. "The Protocols of the Learned Experts on Heroin." *The Libertarian Review,* July 1981.

———. *Psychiatric Slavery.* Syracuse, N.Y.: Syracuse University Press, 1977.

———. *Psychiatry: The Science of Lies.* Syracuse, N.Y.: Syracuse University Press, 2008.

———. "The Sane Slave: Social Control and Legal Psychiatry." *American Criminal Law Review* 10, no. 337 (1971–1972).

———. *Schizophrenia: The Sacred Symbol of Psychiatry.* Syracuse, N.Y.: Syracuse University Press, 1988 [1976].

———. *The Theology of Medicine: The Political-Philosophical Foundations of Medical Ethics.* Syracuse, N.Y.: Syracuse University Press, 1988 [1977].

———. *The Therapeutic State: Psychiatry in the Mirror of Current Events.* Buffalo, N.Y.: Prometheus Books, 1984.

Talcott, Selden Haines. "Freedom in Medical Matters." *New York Times* letter to the editor, February 24, 1891, p. 3.

———. "Hahnemann and His Influence upon Modern Medicine." An Address Delivered at the Homoeopathic Festival, Boston, April 12, 1887. Place of publication not identified, 1887. Available online at HathiTrust Digital Library.

———. *Mental Diseases and their Modern Treatment.* Middletown, N.Y.: Sagwan Press, 2015.

———. "New Methods in the Treatment of the Insane." *North American Journal of Homeopathy* XLIX (1901): 528–31.

Treuherz, Francis, and Sylvain Cazalet, presenters. "Hospitals and Sanatoriums of the Homoeopathic School of Medicine." Homéopathe International (website).

Turner, Justin G., and Linda Levitt Turner, eds. *Mary Todd Lincoln: Her Life and Letters.* New York: Alfred A. Knopf, 1972.

Van der Post, Sietse T., et al. "Strong Frequency Dependence of Vibrational Relaxation in Bulk and Surface Water Reveals Sub-picosecond Structural Heterogeneity." Nature Communications 6 (2015): 8384.

von Boenninghausen, Clemens Maria Franz. *The Lesser Writings of C. M. F. von Boenninghausen.* London: Forgotten Books, 2018.

———. *Boenninghausen's Therapeutic Pocket-Book for Homeopathic Physicians: To Use at the Bedside and in the Study of the Materia Medica.* Franklin Classics Trade Press, 2018.

Walach, H. "Entanglement Model of Homeopathy as an Example of Generalized Entanglement Predicted by Weak Quantum Theory." *Forsch Komplementarmed Klass Naturheilkd* (October 2003): 192–200.

Whitaker, Robert. *Anatomy of an Epidemic: Magic Bullets, Psychiatric Drugs, and the Astonishing Rise of Mental Illness in America.* New York: Broadway Books, 2015.

———. *Mad in America: Bad Science, Bad Medicine, and the Enduring Mistreatment of the Mentally Ill.* New York: Perseus, 2010.

———. "Polypharmacy/Bipolar Illness." MadinAmerica.com, November 22, 2011.

Wilson, Jacquelyn J., M. D., and Forrest J. Murphy, eds. *Anthology: 150 Years of the American Institute of Homeopathy.* St. Louis, Mo.: Formur Incorporated Publishers, 1994.

Winston, Julian. "Influenza–1918: Homeopathy to the Rescue." *The New England Journal of Homeopathy* 7, no. 1, Spring/Summer 1998.

Worcester, Samuel. *Insanity and Its Treatment. Lectures on the Treatment of Insanity and Kindred Nervous Diseases.* New York and Philadelphia: Boericke & Tafel, 1882.

Yanni, Carla. *The Architecture of Madness: Insane Asylums in the United States.* Minneapolis: University of Minnesota Press, 2007.

Young, Sue. *The Wesselhoeft Family and Homeopathy,* 2007. SueYoungHistories .com.

Zhang, J. M., and J. An. "Cytokines, Inflammation, and Pain. *Int Anesthesiol Clin.* 45, no. 2 (2007): 27–37.

# Index

# About the Author

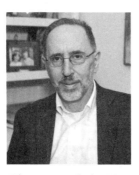

Jerry M. Kantor is the author of four other books: *Interpreting Chronic Illness: The Convergence of Traditional Chinese Medicine, Homeopathy, and Biomedicine; The Toxic Relationship Cure: Clearing Traumatic Damage from a Boss, Parent, Lover, or Friend with Natural, Drug-free Remedies; Autism Reversal Toolbox: Strategies, Remedies, Resources;* and under the pseudonym Chaim Yankel, *Heymischer Homeopathy, the Schmendrick's Guide to Remedying Yiddish Kvetches.* He holds a B.A. in philosophy from Queens College, CUNY; a master's in the management of human services from Brandeis University; and is a graduate of the Advanced Acupuncture Program for Foreign Students, Nanjing College of Traditional Medicine, People's Republic of China.

Kantor's Boston-area acupuncture and homeopathy practice specializes in pediatrics, mental illness, autism spectrum ailments, autoimmune conditions, and infertility. He lectures and teaches across North America and is a faculty member of the Ontario College of Homeopathic Medicine. He was the first acupuncturist granted an academic appointment at Harvard Medical School's Department of Anaesthesiology. A longtime practitioner of qi gong and tai qi, Kantor holds a fourth-degree black belt in the Japanese martial art aikido.